'This book is a posthumous gift from Tom Andersen, sensitively edited and compiled by colleagues who knew the man and his work. It is a vitally important volume for anyone continuing to strive to make their practice a mutually humanising process. Tom Andersen movingly elaborates on the history of those ideas and people who inspired and sometimes challenged him. He takes the reader through each step of his professional life, and his continuing search to find peace in his work and peace of mind in his practice together with others.

This is a joy to read and a warm reminder of a man who really knew how to listen. Some years ago, Tom said to me, "Listen to your wisdom". There is much wisdom in the lines of this book that will continue to inspire those open to listening and learning from one of Family Therapy's greatest pioneers.'

Jim Wilson, *Independent Systemic Consultant, Author and Trainer*

Wanderings and Crossroads

Wanderings and Crossroads: Touch and Participation in Psychiatry and Other Peace Work is made up of three unfinished manuscripts that Andersen was working on at the time of his death, deftly and expertly brought together by the volume editors, and published here in English for the first time.

Tom Andersen continues to have a huge influence on the systemic and family therapy field, and on mental health professions more broadly. This unique volume follows on from Andersen's previous work with his renowned team in Tromsø, presenting the vital work they conducted. This book offers Andersen's personal history and his development as a doctor and psychiatrist, in his own words, offering a theoretical, practical and autoethnographic insight into this pioneering figure.

This book invites readers into the practical and conceptual world of Tom Andersen and will be of interest to those involved in individual, family, group and network therapy and counselling.

Tom Andersen was Professor of Social Psychiatry at the Institute of Community Medicine, University of Tromsø, Norway, and was the pioneer of reflective processes in therapeutic practices.

Magnus Hald is a Senior Consultant Psychiatrist at the Medication Free Treatment Unit, University Hospital of North Norway.

Bengt Karlsson is a Professor Emeritus at the University of South-Eastern Norway, Norway.

Rolf Sundet is a Professor Emeritus at the University of South-Eastern Norway, Norway.

The Systemic Thinking and Practice Series
Series Editors: Charlotte Burck and Gwyn Daniel

This influential series was co-founded in 1989 by series editors David Campbell and Ros Draper to promote innovative applications of systemic theory to psychotherapy, teaching, supervision and organisational consultation. In 2011, Charlotte Burck and Gwyn Daniel became series editors and aim to present new theoretical developments and pioneering practice, to make links with other theoretical approaches, and to promote the relevance of systemic theory to contemporary social and psychological questions.

Recent titles in the series include:

Psychotherapeutic Competencies
Techniques, Relationships, and Epistemology in Systemic Practice
Laura Fruggeri, Francesca Balestra and Elena Venturelli

Systemic Perspectives in Mental Health, Social Work and Youth Care
Anke Savenije, Justine van Lawick and Ellen Reijmers

Systemic and Narrative Work with Unaccompanied Asylum-Seeking Children
Stories of Relocation
Ana Draper, Elisa Marcellino and Samantha Thomson

Systemic-Dialogical Therapy with Individuals
Finding One's Place
Paolo Bertrando and Claudia Lini

Wanderings and Crossroads
Touch and Participation in Psychiatry and Other Peace Work
Tom Andersen, Edited by Magnus Hald, Bengt Karlsson and Rolf Sundet

Wanderings and Crossroads

Touch and Participation in Psychiatry and Other Peace Work

Tom Andersen

Edited by Magnus Hald,
Bengt Karlsson and Rolf Sundet

Routledge
Taylor & Francis Group
LONDON AND NEW YORK

First published in English 2026 by Routledge

First published 2026
by Routledge
4 Park Square, Milton Park, Abingdon, Oxon OX14 4RN

and by Routledge
605 Third Avenue, New York, NY 10158

Routledge is an imprint of the Taylor & Francis Group, an informa business

Translated by Deep L Pro

For Product Safety Concerns and Information please contact our EU representative GPSR@taylorandfrancis.com. Taylor & Francis Verlag GmbH, Kaufingerstraße 24, 80331 München, Germany.

Published in Norwegian (Bokmål) by Vigmostad & Bjørke AS, 2021

British Library Cataloguing-in-Publication Data
A catalogue record for this book is available from the British Library

ISBN: 978-1-032-41365-5 (hbk)
ISBN: 978-1-032-41364-8 (pbk)
ISBN: 978-1-003-35774-2 (ebk)

DOI: 10.4324/9781003357742

Typeset in Times New Roman
by codeMantra

Contents

Series editors' foreword ix
Foreword by Harlene Anderson xi
Foreword xiv

Introduction 1

An introduction to this book's content and context 6

PART 1
Professional and historical walks 15

1 Tom Andersen: lived life, democracy and contexts 17

2 Historical walks 21

PART 2
Professional crossroads 29

3 The first experiments and steps 31

4 The next experiments and steps 50

5 About reflective teams and processes 71

PART 3
The place and importance of language 89

6 The power of words – yes, the power of expressions 91

7 The meanings of expressions in treatment and research 104

PART 4
Descriptions from different practices 129

8 Descriptions of collaborating practices with patients, families and networks 131

9 Four practices where language and conversations are central 139

10 Shared context, shared history and shared culture – practices in the North Calotte 151

References *185*
Appendices: Tom Andersen's bibliography collected and edited by Petter H. Næsje *190*
Afterword *199*
Index *203*

Series editors' foreword

Wanderings and Crossroads. A book about touch and participation in psychiatry and other peace work. Tom Andersen. Edited by Magnus Hald, Bengt Karlsson and Rolf Sundet

When Magnus Hald, Bengt Karlsson and Rolf Sundet let us know that they were the inheritors of unpublished writings by Tom Andersen, which they were editing into a book, we were immediately intrigued.

Tom Andersen and the team in Tromsø transformed our systemic field through their development of the reflecting team, a model which he presented at many international conferences and which is articulated in his paper, The reflecting team: dialogue and meta-dialogue in clinical work (Family Process 1987) and his book, *The Reflecting Team: Dialogues and Dialogues about Dialogues* (Norton 1991). The use of the reflecting team and of reflecting processes in general has since been adapted in many different contexts worldwide and continues to be incorporated into current practices. However, despite being renowned throughout the systemic world, Tom Andersen published relatively few articles in his lifetime.

What a privilege, therefore, to be able to have access to previously undiscovered writing of Tom Andersen, incomplete as they were, due to his untimely death.

We learnt from the three Norwegian editors how little Tom Andersen's work in the mental health field has been valued by the Norwegian psychiatric profession, despite his worldwide reputation. It was in this traditional and rather critical context that Tom developed his thinking and practice, drawing our attention to how brave and radical he was.

One of the most valuable aspects of this book, edited together by his three colleagues, lies in the detail Tom Andersen provides of the processes of his learning. It is rare to have a clinician identify and track the experimentations involved in learning from doing and to follow the opportunities that present themselves along the way. This book allows us to accompany him as he works out what he thinks, what he senses would be worth exploring and what would not be, while all the time trying to pay close attention to feedback from families, from other professionals and from himself. He dares to take non-traditional, non-conforming pathways as he steps into new territories, where sometimes the learning is painful.

Many readers will be familiar with Tom Andersen's work in broad brush strokes – almost everybody will know of the facilitative approaches of reflecting teams and processes, and many too will know a few phrases for which Tom became known – "if your fist could speak on the way to hit, what would it say?" (1991), which bridged the embodied and linguistic components of communication. There has been less opportunity to follow his process of thinking and the ways in which he developed his collaboration with family members through his careful attention to feedback. Here, besides descriptions of his wandering professional routes, he gives us vivid extracts from his therapy sessions, having watched some recordings of sessions over and over again. These clinical extracts bring Tom Andersen, and the family members and professionals with whom he worked, very much to life, and, as qualitative evidence so often does, show us ways to work towards attentive collaborations.

We are very pleased to have this book in our series, which we think will be highly valued by our systemic community.

Charlotte Burck, Gwyn Daniel and Lizette Nolte

Foreword by Harlene Anderson

I was honoured when asked to write a foreword for this book. My first thought was what a daunting task. My second thought was what would Tom hope I would say, and what would be helpful for the reader? Someone once told me that they found forewords helpful that let the reader know something about the author. Throughout the book, you have the opportunity to know Tom through his own words. I thought I knew Tom fairly well, but this book offered the privilege to learn more about Tom from his own words, particularly his thinking processes and what influenced them. As Tom said of himself, he was a *wanderer*. I would say he was an *intellectual wanderer* and *risk-taker*. Most impressively, he was a fearless challenger of the status quo, especially regarding social justice and inequality issues. Every time I met him, I wondered what would he bring with him that would inspire me to reflect on who I think I am with others.

Tom's last words at the end of this book capture the gift he left for us and the people we meet in our daily lives as he spoke of the ultimate influence we can have for those we meet and for ourselves: "Conflicts and tensions will diminish, and the therapist will become less wilful and less easily caught up in their own feelings and experiences of the situation, the clients and themselves".

I first met Tom decades ago at one of the early team conferences in Europe. At that time, I didn't initiate interaction with him and his colleague. Following the team meeting, Tom invited Harry to Norway to participate in his June summer school. Harry returned with rave reviews of the experience and Tom. The next year, Tom invited both Harry and me to his summer school. We travelled to Norway with Harry's wife and my husband. We were there for about a month, starting in Oslo and travelling, providing workshops and meeting many people from the far south of Norway to Northern Norway. Early in our trip, on the coast far south, we were surprised to hear that we were going to a research conference. One of the first lessons learnt. A word does not necessarily mean what you think it does or sounds like. People were talking about a small town whose name sounded like research to our Texas ears. On the way back to the hotel, we discussed the surprising news about a research conference and simply decided that we would figure out what to do when we got there. I mention this because it fits with one of the themes that runs throughout this book: in my words, life is full of surprises, and you cannot fully know beforehand what it will be and how you will respond. We were confident we would be able to respond in the moment; we could not know ahead of time.

Another stop was a visit with a psychiatrist in historic Narvik, Norway, who Tom said we must meet. Harry and our host stayed up all night talking. The plans were to drive further north to meet more mental health professionals. Tired, Harry and our host got in the back seat of the car, handed me the keys and said, "We want you to drive". Dumbfounded, I asked where to and how would I know how to get there. Our host confidently said, "Once you're on the road, you can only go north". And off to sleep they went. Once I found the highway, I drove for hours on various roads and through several seemingly never-ending tunnels and saw striking glacier-formed vistas of mountains and fjords. This was an amazing experience, which I later thought of as what might be an example of the relational two-way aspect of trust. I trusted these two men who trusted and had confidence in me.

We eventually met up again with Tom in a tiny Norwegian town to meet the local doctor, a character who wore shiny red patent leather shoes. Little did I know this Norwegian excursion was the beginning of a sustained friendship and collaboration with Tom and his creative colleagues. Though most of the trip was an experience of not-knowing, importantly, it was an experience in the value of maintaining relationships with colleagues no matter how far or near. And, that we can learn as much or more from the people we serve and our colleagues as we can learn from academically acclaimed masters.

As a reader, you are highly fortunate to eavesdrop and imagine you are hearing Tom's voice. It was a privilege for me to read his words and to be moved by his descriptions of some of the paths he took and the influences of his personal and professional journeys. Tom's sharing of his life experiences is a good reminder for all of us that we are not merely professionals performing our roles, but we are human beings with varied experiences. From Tom and his colleagues, I experienced and learnt the value of respect, of having patience and tentativeness, and of the potential of the phrase "it might be". This reminds me of the importance of congruency in our various roles as human beings. You, the reader, are privileged to meet Tom as the person he shows us on these pages and his passionate alliance to living his values. None of us will ever fully know Tom or any other person. This book, however, provides a glimpse into his inner thoughts.

What sustained this mutually influential friendship-colleagueship? Firstly, I highlight Tom's respect for people, no matter what their status as simply human beings. Closely related are his high regard for the knowledge and wisdom each person has for their own life that they bring to our encounters and his ability to discard the professional illusion and intent that we can change another person. I remember Tom once warning of the importance of how our histories and contexts influence how we experience another person and interpret their words. He continued, suggesting how through our ideas and interactions, we participate in creating the person in front of us, and of course, inviting their responses to us. My colleague Harry Goolishian once said to me, "Harlene, you cannot change another person, you can only change yourself." I agree; however, this is a challenging task for most of us.

Perhaps believing and trusting this is the first challenge. Tom agreed. I hope I will always remember this and the wisdom Tom shares in this book.

Tom would be modestly pleased that the manuscripts he left behind might inspire many of us to similarly be the kind of reflective-reflexive practitioner he was, taking the time to pause, step back, and critically reflect on our experiences, and the usefulness of what we have learnt from our experiences can continue to be beneficial as we continue forward. I hope that as you reflect on and interact with Tom's words, stories and realities he shares on these pages, you will feel you have met or revisited the sceptical and hopeful person Tom was. He inspired me to think, and hopefully you as well. May you leave with the sense that, as Tom suggests, language is a social and relational activity through which we create and live our realities.

Harlene Anderson
Houston, Texas U.S.
June 2025

Foreword

It was with awe and excitement that we three editors of this book embarked on the work. First and foremost, because this book, as it now stands, is made up of three manuscripts that Tom Andersen himself probably did not consider to be finished. They were works in progress and constantly changing in line with his own work and his thoughts and encounters with different environments and people. The joy and enthusiasm quickly grew as we worked on the scripts and realised how they were connected in both form and content. And, not least, how the texts are highly relevant to clinical practice, research and education. We hope that we have managed to do justice to Tom Andersen and the three manuscripts he left behind when he died in 2007. For us, it has been an honour to work with these texts, and we believe that they hold great value in our time, both nationally and internationally.

First and foremost, we would like to thank the family of Siri Andersen, Sjur Andersen, Simen Hofgaard Andersen and Sille Hofgaard Andersen for giving their permission for Fagbokforlaget to publish the texts. We would also like to thank Petter Næsje, who has generously shared his knowledge and a complete bibliography of Tom Andersen's works. We would also like to thank Fagbokforlaget, represented by editor Nikolai Fjeld, who enthusiastically demonstrated his belief in the project through his friendly consultation during the work.

Tromsø/Oslo/Drammen

Magnus Hald, Bengt Karlsson and Rolf Sundet

Introduction

When Tom Andersen died in May 2007 after an accident, he left behind three unfinished book manuscripts. Magnus Hald succeeded in preserving them. The book you are now holding in your hands is based on these three manuscripts, which totalled around 600 A4 pages. We have processed, edited and selected from them so that they provide a coherent expression in the form of this book.

Reading through the manuscripts, it becomes clear that Tom Andersen's ambition was for the three manuscripts to result in three independent book publications. The title of this book is composed of the titles of two of the manuscripts. The first – *Wanderings and Crossroads* – describes Tom Andersen's personal and professional wanderings. Through various professional contexts as a doctor, and later as a social psychiatrist and family therapist, he portrays how his thinking and understanding changes and points to new paths to follow. In his manuscript *Touch and Participation in Psychiatry and Other Peace Work*, he emphasises the understanding and importance of the body, breath, words and being touched by one's own and others' impressions and expressions. In addition, he describes how the work in the mental health field is about dialogue and collaboration with people, like what happens in diplomacy, peace work and ordinary life. The third manuscript deals with collaboration in the North Calotte between Swedish, Finnish and Norwegian colleagues – and later also professionals from Russia. Andersen was keen to ensure that this co-operation was rooted in the area's history, culture and nature.

The book you now hold in your hands is mainly based on the first two manuscripts and, to a lesser extent, the last one on the North Calotte. A shortened version of the manuscript on the North Calotte co-operation can be found in the last chapter of this book. When we started processing and editing the three manuscripts, they had not been fully produced or edited by Andersen. His ambition was to outline how his own professional development and changes from 1964 to 2007 could be described. When editing the manuscripts, we had to create our own titles for all parts and chapters of the book, precisely because it is based on three manuscripts. The intertitles and subtitles are based on Andersen's three manuscripts. This Introduction and the Afterword is written by us, the three editors. All other text is original work written by Tom Andersen. In the surviving manuscripts, Tom Andersen's own lived experiences are highly significant for the collaborations he developed and participated in

DOI: 10.4324/9781003357742-1

various parts of the world. In a text he calls "The curse of oppression; a source of democracy", he shows how a seminal experience from his childhood influenced his work and ideas about collaboration with other people throughout his life and work.

It was 2021, and we began editing this book. Fifteen years have passed since Andersen described his thoughts and work as an expression of a naivety that was, and is, important to maintain. The last 15 years have shown in different ways that the world needs more openness, more co-operation, more sharing through listening and being moved at all levels – individually, in communities, in nations and in the world at large. We believe that the ideas and, not least, the practices that Tom Andersen, together with his colleagues, developed and worked with, stand up very well, as the world still needs them. His basic ideas and assumptions are both simple and complex, and they still apply today. Take his idea that no one can be changed from the outside. People can only be invited to change. If someone pressurises or forces someone to change, resistance and opposition develop. We see several examples of the latter among individuals, groups, populations and countries that are forced to make changes with dramatic consequences for them. Tom Andersen himself exemplified this with various forms of dictatorship, disregard for human rights and the use of force in treatment.

Against this background, Andersen describes his activities as work against oppression. He quotes Martin Luther King, who said, "Peace is not the absence of conflict, but the presence of justice". Andersen describes his understanding of peace work as the effort and work in which all people in a situation, in a family, in a local community and in society should have the same basic right to express themselves and be heard. No one should be threatened or silenced. This is the fundamental idea of democracy and of the peace work that is carried out in families, networks, local communities and in war. No voice should be prioritised and allowed to dominate, and no voice should be silenced or suppressed.

Tom Andersen's practice and understanding of research also changed significantly through his work with families, people in prison and the use of coercion in mental health care. His first research work was in the field of biological psychiatry and related to neuroleptic depot medication. He completed his doctorate in social psychiatry in 1978 with a comparative study of psychiatric morbidity in two municipalities in Northern Norway. Andersen later described how his doctorate enabled him to take up a position at the university. This gave him the opportunity to explore new and different avenues to a greater extent than would have been possible in an ordinary clinical position. This was how Andersen became interested in the connection between body and mind through his collaboration with psychomotor therapists Gudrun Øvreberg and Aadel Bülow-Hansen. He brought this knowledge into conversations and meetings with people as individuals, families and larger systems. When Andersen became interested and involved in family therapy and systemic thinking and practice, he was inspired by the work of key professionals such as Jay Haley and Salvador Minuchin. He collaborated with the Milan Group, particularly Gianfranco Cecchin, and with Peggy Penn and Lynn Hoffmann and extensively with Harlene Anderson, Harry Goolishian and John Shotter. Inspired by the aforementioned, as well as by colleagues in Tromsø, the idea of "the reflective team and processes" was born and developed. This was an innovation in systemic practice and family therapy, and later also in several other contexts where people collaborated on something and with someone. Everything about reflective teams and processes contributed to Tom Andersen gaining an international arena, while international conferences and seminars were created in Northern Norway for the benefit of Norwegian and Scandinavian colleagues. This work led Andersen to meetings with Jaakko Seikkula, among others. Together with the latter and Norwegian, Swedish, Finnish and Russian colleagues, the North Calotte co-operation was launched. This involved educational programmes, seminars and research projects. Until Tom Andersen's death, he was active in all these areas. He also co-operated with people with developmental disabilities and individuals who were incarcerated. All these meetings with national and international professionals inspired, challenged and developed him as both a professional and a human being.

Tom Andersen emphasises his own wanderings in the professional landscape. He shows how his wanderings interacted with him as a person and shaped the life he lived. His professional orientation was a continuous process of change, characterised by his creativity and desire to challenge conventions and professional boundaries. He was uncompromising and highly critical of psychiatry, both as a profession and as a health service, an attitude that led him through many new stages. His occasional uncompromising and critical attitude may, for some, have made him difficult to follow. Andersen himself emphasises that it is important for him to use the term "crossroads" rather than "fork in the road". His professional development, growth and change followed their own paths. Andersen points out that there were many crossroads in his professional journey and the connections between them are just as important as their number. He describes how the crossroads are interconnected and can be expressed in a more abbreviated version. Andersen shows how the crossroads have developed both historically and in line with the development of his professional journeys. He describes the fork in the road, from either-or to both-and, as follows:

> There was a big shift from "either-or" to "both-and". Without realising it at the time, I would now say that "either-or" belongs to a world that can be described as motionless, and you could say "the non-living". In other words, we were working with living people who belonged to the "non-living". It felt uncomfortable, and it was a relief to move on to "both-and". But we also had to leave the closed room - it was uncomfortable to be there.
>
> (Jensen, 2008, p. 193)

Andersen argues that both-and was a reckoning with the closed space, along with an understanding of the body and the importance of seeing and listening to the bodies in the room. Andersen describes how the physiotherapist Bülow-Hansen strongly influenced him through the way she used her eyes and, importantly, how she listened. Andersen emphasises:

> When you look and listen, you experience it through your body, and then something happens in your body. First you feel it with your body, then you feel it in your body - and then come the expressions, and with the expressions come the meanings.

This understanding of the relationship between impressions and expressions is also reflected in the framework of reflective processes. Tom Andersen writes that the principle is simple; when the listening team receives the story the family wants them to hear, the team is usually moved by it. What happens to them when they are moved, for example, by an idea, a question or a feeling, is passed back to the family. The story touches the listener, and the listener returns what happened to him or her.

In 1996, colleagues of Tom Andersen wrote:

> Tom has a strong and distinctive personality that no one can be indifferent to, and in Norwegian psychiatry he has been, and is, a colourful troublemaker. It's been tough at times, but he enjoys it the most. Since the mid-1980s, he has been increasingly recognised as a leader in family therapy and systemic thinking and practice, both nationally and internationally. Today, he is by far the most internationally recognised Norwegian psychiatrist in the field of family therapy.
>
> (University of Tromsø, 1996)

In a later interview, Andersen says:

> I've often been afraid. Especially afraid of being ridiculed and laughed at in public, and I certainly have been. And then, of course, I'm afraid of hurting people, but that's not what I've been most afraid of. I hear that in parts of Norwegian psychiatry I have a so-called "non-name". It's not a very pleasant thing to hear.
>
> (Jensen, 2008, p. 206)

We believe that the publication of this book re-emphasises the importance of Tom Andersen's thoughts, ideas and practices, and, not least, the reputation he still holds in Norway, Scandinavia, Europe and the rest of the world. We believe that Andersen has put to shame the notion that he is a "non-name" in Norwegian psychiatry. There is hardly any other Norwegian psychiatrist who has had such impact and significance in mental health work, both nationally and internationally, as Tom Andersen. We thought it might be appropriate to reproduce excerpts from what Professor Per Jensen wrote in his eulogy to Tom Andersen, entitled "Solidarity":

> Tom gave it his all. He wanted to touch, to connect. It seemed as if he was addicted to getting in touch. No contact, no teaching. For Tom, teaching

a small group of students was just as important as presentations at large international congresses, there was no difference. His demands on himself to reach hearts meant the same whether there were three students at Diakonhjemmet or many hundreds at a conference. Tom was faithful, faithful to his friends. He never cancelled a lesson. Nothing ever got in the way. The money he earned from his book *Reflective Processes* and from his presentations went in its entirety to someone who needed it more than he did. To his friends. They were in the north, in the east and in the south. He was generous to those who didn't have much. Tom could build networks. Tom could participate in networks. Tom could contribute to networks. This has left a lasting impression, for example in the Arctic and South America (...) Tom was uncompromising when it came to using human-friendly language. He avoided anything that evoked an understanding of reality that is used in descriptions of the mechanical world, and he recommended that we do the same. Words like "technique" and "method" are examples of what for him were such mechanical descriptions (...) I know what I see when I look into the word "solidarity". I see Tom.

(Jensen, 2008, pp. 252–253)

Tom Andersen represented a major and important challenge to the prevailing scepticism about methods, techniques and traditional diagnostic systems. Despite resistance, he uncompromisingly followed his own path. He helped create a more open space with opportunities for new conversations while also presenting alternatives. Andersen's work has created major ripple effects. A very interesting aspect of his practice is that it can be used in many different contexts, including cultural and political ones. He was a very patient therapist, yet at the same time impatient with the inertia of the structures of society. In this area, he gave, and still gives, challenges to Norwegian and international professionals.

We hope that this book does full justice to the professional Tom Andersen was, and still is, through his thoughts, videos, books and articles. Justice, in the sense that Andersen was far more professionally respected in Scandinavia, Europe, Latin America, Japan and the USA than in the Norwegian professional tradition of psychiatry and his own professional group of psychiatrists. In the Norwegian environments, he was rarely mentioned or met with respect and curiosity by his own profession. Andersen's thinking and working methods spread internationally, and he was invited to give presentations, teach and mentor in several places around the world. As a result, he met numerous professionals who became partners, and he was part of various national and international networks from the mid-1970s onwards, many of which are still going strong after Tom Andersen's death in 2007. His collaboration with physiotherapists greatly contributed to thinking about the connections between breath, tension and words. Within the conversational part of his work, it is mentioned how inspiration from the family therapy tradition contributed to new thinking and new practices. We hope that this book brings renewed life and excitement to Andersen, his ideas and work, and that it inspires further development of these practices and ideas.

An introduction to this book's content and context

In this introduction, we tie together parts of what we described in the introduction about the person Tom Andersen, the manuscripts he left behind and how his work and ways of thinking have inspired many professionals across the world. What follows is an introductory deep dive into key ideas and practices developed by Andersen. The three of us who are editing the book also write about how we came to know Andersen, his work and how it has inspired us as professionals. Overall, this book is an invitation to get to know Tom Andersen's thoughts, conceptualisations and practices related to (co-)working with families and their networks within what was previously referred to as "psychiatry", now called mental health care. Why work with families and eventually their networks? The 1940s and 1950s saw the emergence of forms of therapy that increasingly included family members. There were many reasons for this. During this period, there was an increasing focus on the conditions in which children and young people grew up. Psychoanalysis had a particular focus on childhood, which in turn led to an increased focus on adolescence. In addition, there were observations from psychiatric hospitals where the patient, after being discharged to the family, relapsed or where others in the family developed symptoms and illness after the patient's return home. As a doctor at Åsgård Hospital in Tromsø, Tom Andersen gained experience by travelling out of the hospital and meeting partners and patients at home. He observed that patients behaved differently in the home setting compared to the hospital environment. This contributed to Andersen becoming aware of the importance of context and adopting a more contextual perspective when working with patients at Åsgård Hospital.

In this work, as in all new treatment work, new challenges were encountered. Imagine two different situations. First, you are a health or social worker in an individual counselling session where the patient is talking about his or her relationship with a parent, father or mother. Imagine a different situation in which you are leading a conversation where everyone in the family is present and the patient is talking about their relationship with mum or dad. These will be experienced as two different situations with different challenges, and in the family conversation, you are faced with a phenomenon where what is said about someone else who is present will lead to immediate reactions, positive or negative, depending on what is said. Furthermore, what happens between the two has effects and causes reactions from

DOI: 10.4324/9781003357742-2

the others in the room. This is a situation that poses completely different challenges for the health and social care worker than if they were talking to the patient alone.

What quickly became clear to those working in family counselling and family therapy was that completely new ways of thinking about problems, treatment, therapist roles and skills were needed. This required new ways of talking and understanding. Central to this was how to describe, talk about and understand interactions between people in the here-and-now situation, including what the therapist should do. To cut a long story short, this was aided by scientific approaches known as information theory, communication theory, cybernetics and systems theory.

During the 1950s, 1960s and 1970s, several forms of family therapy developed that focused on interaction and communication between family members and between them and the therapist, using language inspired and influenced by the above-mentioned theories. One such method, developed in Italy in the 1970s and further developed in the early 1980s, was the Milan method, or systemic family therapy. A distinctive feature was that several therapists worked together in the family counselling sessions, with one or two were with the family and two or more sitting behind a one-way mirror. They saw and heard what was happening in the room where one worked with the family. At some point, the therapist(s) who were in the room with the family left and went to the room behind the mirror to confer with their colleagues, after which an intervention in the form of a message was created for the family.

Tom Andersen worked in Tromsø with colleagues and was inspired and influenced by the development of various family therapies. In this book, you will find his descriptions of these sources of inspiration and what they meant for his work. At one point, something decisive happened. Instead of the therapist who was with the family going behind the mirror and creating an intervention, the sound and light were turned around so that the family and the therapists could listen to and observe the conversation behind the mirror. The team's thoughts, ideas and reflections were now made available to the family. The book documents that this was experienced as a radical and revolutionary change for the professionals involved, and suddenly the reflective team was born.

In many ways, the birth of the reflective team can be seen as being in language and conversation, and, as the book shows, the importance of conversation and how it is conducted. The sources of inspiration for this development are clearly shown in the book to be the meeting and collaboration with Harry Goolishian. Goolishian, together with Harlene Anderson, represented a shift in the field of family therapy away from systems, cybernetics and communication models and towards a focus on language and conversation. In the book, you will find several descriptions of conversations with families and reflections on what a good conversation entails. In this work, we believe there is a shift in Tom Andersen's way of thinking about his work, which is perhaps his most original contribution to the field of family therapy. Working with and in reflective teams and what eventually became known as reflective processes can, from the texts that make up this book, be seen as an amalgam of influences from different theoretical and practical perspectives. More importantly, this amalgam is made up of inputs, contributions and influences from all the different professional groups and individuals with whom Tom, over many years, worked, and who must be credited with a share in the development of reflective teams and processes.

The distinctive and potentially timeless

The uniqueness that we believe Tom brings also has its sources of inspiration. These are the works of Aadel Bülow-Hansen and Gudrun Øvreberg in the field of physiotherapy. By working with them, the importance of the body, breathing and movement comes into play. The focus is no longer on the linguistic meaning but on what it is in the speech that reveals, via the body's reactions, what the individual is affected by in their own speech. The body's reactions to one's own speech become a guide to what one can touch on in the conversation. This is what can be called the affective turn in family therapy and what we believe is one of Tom Andersen's most crucial contributions. Two things stand out. Firstly, perhaps paradoxically, every event, phenomenon, characteristic or aspect of life is given an understanding through its contextual and historical location. The paradox lies in the fact that this statement clearly has its contextual location. This is the medical specialty of psychiatry's approach to and perspective on mental illness or disease. Psychiatric illness is dealt with through diagnoses that are context-independent and where the treatment is method-specific and person-independent. If you have a diagnosis and a method that has been scientifically tested, currently through research using the randomised control design, then the people, be it the patient or the therapist, are uninteresting. They can be replaced because the connection between diagnosis and method is precisely context- and person-independent. Tom Andersen was clearly an opponent of this perspective and, as such, a controversial figure in his own professional group. This was not where he primarily found support and inspiration. Tom never hid the fact that he was a doctor and psychiatrist, but in his own way.

The other area that is context-independent and timeless, in the sense that it is always with us, is ethics. At the same time, these ethics are always directed towards the person and the context they are part of. Throughout Tom's work, we find a preoccupation with and involvement in ethics, not ethics as a set of rules, but ethics as the question we all face in our encounters with others: How should I behave so that both the other person and I do not deteriorate? The other person knows what I am inflicting on them and on myself precisely by inflicting something that is painful, wrong, unpleasant and/or disrespectful to the other person. In other words, ethics is about how each of us emerges as a subject in the encounter with the other. Furthermore, the answer to this question does not lie in rules and ethical theories but in the response you get from the other person. How is the other person affected by what I say and do? Ultimately, this is perhaps the most decisive aspect of Tom's work: a continuous preoccupation with how each of us can take care of the relationship with the other and the other in this relationship. This is where we find the subtitle he has given us for this book: touch and participation in psychiatry and other peace work.

The editors' approach to this book's content

In 1988, while Bengt was undertaking further training in psychiatric nursing, he came across a book chapter written by the Norwegian psychiatrist Tom Andersen. The chapter was titled "Change knows its own time and its own way" (Andersen, 1987). In it, Andersen and his colleagues introduced the practical importance of change, language and co-operation. For Bengt, reading this chapter was a revelation and the beginning lifelong exploration, both theoretical and practical, of what it meant to (co-)work with change and language in an ethical and reflexive sense. Andersen's basic ethical stance and imperative, developed in the 1980s and remained until his death in 2008, can be summarised as follows: "Listen to people's experiences and believe in what they say. Ethics and dialogue come first. Talk to people and not about. If I think people can't bear to hear what I have to say, keep your mouth shut".

Magnus met Tom as a medical student at the University of Tromsø in 1978. He was interested in psychiatry as a discipline even before he started studying and was particularly interested in psychodynamic thinking and practice based on psychodynamic ideas. Tom represented a challenging and ultimately fascinating alternative. He argued in favour of a contextual understanding and the importance of meeting those who wanted help from such a perspective. He showcased his own practice in a very different way from other teachers: both using video and role-playing and by giving interested parties extensive opportunities to join him in clinical practice. In conversations with individuals and families, Tom was present in a very special way. He had an ability to listen so that everyone felt understood. After completing his internship, Magnus started working as a doctor at Åsgård Hospital, where Tom was a consultant in a secondary position. There, he worked closely with Tom and other colleagues on developing work with reflective teams and reflective processes. The close collaboration with Tom continued until his death in 2007.

Rolf met Tom through the Norwegian Association for Family Therapy around 1985. He was a newly qualified psychologist who had written his thesis on Humberto Maturana, a Chilean biologist who at the time was important in the field of family therapy. Maturana always started his lectures by drawing an eye in the top corner of the blackboard to emphasise that every one of us is an observer, and that any description depends on our gaze and perspective. Rolf struggled to find a practical use for this perspective, immersed as he was in traditional psychology. His meeting with Tom, and his descriptions and explanations of the reflective team, were a revelation. The crucial thing in therapy is that we share our gaze and our perspective, not as truth, but precisely as different gazes and perspectives. The possibility of change lies in the fact that sharing brings out differences (which make a difference).

A short journey in Tom Andersen's world of concepts and practices

The following is an outline of the editor's reading and understanding of the work of Tom Andersen and his colleagues. We do not present this as a "true" and "correct" understanding, but rather, in line with the importance of differences, as an offer of a thread and a contrast that the reader can take with him in his reading. The invitation from the editors is for the reader to create their own understanding of this material.

The change

When Andersen and colleagues developed reflective teams and processes (Andersen, 1987) in the mid-1980s, it was precisely through the "simple" move of turning sound and light around so that the family could listen to what was being said behind the one-way mirror that the importance of differences became clear. The editors claim that this had radical consequences for the practice and understanding of therapeutic work in psychiatry and mental health care.

Using reflective teams, all participants in a conversation are invited to tell their story, switching between speaking and listening positions to give and receive feedback. It is equally important in this approach that professionals acknowledge their feelings and thoughts while all participants are listening. Professionals speak together only when all those involved are present. During the development of this way of working, the professionals in the team found that they had changed. They spoke kindlier to the participants and to each other, and they became keen to ask questions that would elicit as many answers as possible. They became reluctant to make assumptions before meeting people, and they became less concerned with making judgements about participants' statements and actions.

Andersen (1988) describes that the start of the journey towards reflective teams was the desire to change treatment measures related to coercion and control. A group of professionals with an interdisciplinary background met regularly in Tromsø. They read, discussed and video-recorded their own work to understand more about each other's work and how they could develop alternative practices. The concept of change took centre stage, both among the professionals and the people seeking help. Both the concept of change, and how to work with it, became crucial for Andersen and colleagues (1988). The group became preoccupied with Bateson's (1979) phrase about "a difference that makes a difference". This was further developed by the team in Tromsø into a discussion of three types of differences:

1 Those differences that are so small that the person does not notice them,
2 Those differences that are "appropriately" large and lead to a difference and
3 The differences that are too big and do not lead to change.

Replacing the word difference with unusual means that when a person is exposed to something that is too common, they are not invited to change. If the person is exposed to something suitably unusual, the chances of change increase significantly. If the person is exposed to something too unusual, there is no change, but rather rigidity and resistance. For Andersen and colleagues, this understanding of change led them to invite people to talk about things that were suitably unusual for them and in a suitably unusual way. The suitably unusual is the kind of change that doesn't happen in everyday life. This understanding of the relationship between differences and change led the team to work on how to invite people to change(s). Their starting point was that people cannot be changed into just anything. Every one of us has, at any given time, a certain repertoire of possible actions in the face of familiar and unfamiliar situations and experiences. This repertoire can be developed and changed in interaction and conversations with other people. Against this background, the team developed the ideas that people can only be invited to change and that change recognises its own paths. Andersen (1985) writes that controlling and instructive interaction and conversations became impossible. This means that people's development and change cannot be controlled from the outside – they take place from within and can be further developed in meetings and conversations with others. Change can be initiated by ideas that arise in good and respectful relationships. A developing and changing relationship is one that accommodates and freely exchanges different feelings and thoughts about a problem. In this way, the person experiencing the problem can select and use the ideas that they themselves consider to be the best or most useful.

It is based on the above work that we would argue that no one can be changed from the outside. The moment we get ideas about changing the other person, it creates resistance in him or her. Even more challenging is that we objectify the other person. Change is not something we invite; it becomes something we have to instruct or inject. The other person, whom we want to change, becomes a tool in our zeal for change. It is in such situations that we can experience the power of instructive and commanding change to create resistance in us. In this way, resistance helps change, if it is desirable for me, to find its own way. Andersen (1999) refers to two types of change. The first is about restricting what existed beforehand. The change comes from outside and has a controlling, guiding and instructive effect. The second type of change expands or renews what was already there. The only person you can change is yourself. We can all learn but not be taught.

Working together

Tom Andersen (1999) has said that everything we do as professionals – and fellow human beings – is to co-operate, whether we are talking about teaching, research, counselling or treatment. This presupposes that the people involved in the collaboration succeed in working together. Andersen imagined that when collaborating with people who wanted help, it was about the person's desire to change something. Change must, therefore, be understood as something that comes from the person themselves. Change cannot be imposed or take place under the direction of others. This means that the person knows what needs to be changed and how it can best be done, and he or she will know when the change has occurred. According to Andersen, our task as counsellors is then to facilitate the conditions in the collaboration so that the inherent resources of the person seeking help can be used. This is done by recognising that the person is the one with the solution and then working together to find specific contributions that can help.

I demonstrate my attitudes and behaviours through various engaging and collaborative relationships and conversations, whether they are private or personal. My starting point is that I always respond to another person, to what they say or do – I *cannot* not respond. Consequently, I think that my attitude in all professional work or in all forms of human activity should be characterised by collaboration. This work is about us working together to understand, speak, respond and share. All this (collaborative) work takes place in relationships – relationships that enable dialogue, sharing, responding and understanding. The big question is: how can I, as a professional, can invite and facilitate such co-operation? We believe that, regardless of whether the "problem" concerns physical or mental health, financial or social difficulties, a relationship is established between the person or people seeking help and the person or persons who can provide it. This relationship then forms the basis for our co-operation. The most important tool in this collaboration is the conversation or dialogue between the various participants in the collaboration (Andersen, 1999). This applies to life in a family, in social services, in a football team, in a hospital, in a housing association, in a local community, in Europe and in the world. There are two or more people who have to figure out and do "something" together. This "something" is closely linked to how we, who are part of this work, think about each other and how this "something" unfolds in concrete behaviours in the collaboration. Consequently, this collaboration takes on a direction, in health and welfare work, linked to help: How can we collaborate on the help to be provided? We allow ourselves to be involved in the other person's experience of the case, and the other person is similarly involved in our understanding. In this way, we move in an endless spiral of talking together about the issue that engages and moves us. Andersen (1999) refers to the same joint collaboration as expressions that create impressions, and impressions that create expressions. It is an endless spiral of attempts to understand what I understand about the issue and about the other person, and how the other person understands themselves, our relationship and the issue.

It may be that both the person seeking help and the person being helped feel that the chemistry is not right. We don't succeed in working together in a way that develops a relationship and a dialogue. It is in the interpersonal encounter between the helper and the help seeker that the individual user experiences the health and welfare sector and the help provided. The help seeker not only experiences the interpersonal encounter, but also how the framework affects the care provided. This applies to everything from the physical surroundings, their practical and aesthetic design, the opportunities for peace and rest and how and where conversations about private and personal matters are framed (Karlsson & Borg, 2017).

Languages

Language is the best tool we have to reduce misunderstandings and develop mutual understanding through dialogue. At the same time, language can confuse us or make us more unclear and uncertain about what we are trying to express. Andersen (1999) points out that language consists of two main components: the words and the bodily activities that follow the words. The words and the body follow each other and stand in relation to each other. The words refer to both a symbolic and a bodily expression. When a person tells their story, I will «hear" the words by being touched, and get sensory associations by seeing, hearing or tasting the words. If the person uses the word "vomit", this gives me immediate sensory images in the form of smell, colour and texture. This can be followed by a bodily expression that makes me feel unwell. In this way, the word "vomit" becomes part of a bodily activity that takes place between the other person and me and expresses part of our social interaction. Language then appears as a social activity that is created and developed in the relationship. We are focused on both the linguistic expression and the bodily expressions that accompany the words. As co-creators of the dialogue, we pay attention to our own sensory touches and associations, as well as to the bodily activities and expressions.

A person's use of words is not random, in the sense that the words carry a meaning. The meaning is in the word, not underneath or behind it. When a person says that "life is without meaning", this appears to carry meaning in two areas. The person is expressing their perceived and experienced relationship to life, and the meaning life gives the person right there and then. It also expresses the meaning the person experiences of themselves in their life. When the person says this, it can give those who hear the statement meaning, in that they can recognise similar experiences in their own life. This makes it possible to start and conduct a dialogue based on the person's statement. Andersen (1999) emphasises that words come first, then thoughts. The author refers to Goolishian (Anderson & Goolishian, 1988), who said that "It is important to talk so that we can find out what we are thinking". The moment the person tells their story, they will become aware of what they are thinking about their own story. The words that form the story also clarify the person's thoughts and reflections related to the story. The words that are chosen are not chosen at random. The person searches through his or her linguistic repertoire of words to find the one that best expresses his or her thoughts and feelings. When the word or words are found and expressed, the person creates meaning through a clear thought or a vague notion. This underlines the importance of creating linguistic dialogues with the words that can be found between those participating in the dialogue. In the same way as the person, the other participants will look for words that can express their experiences related to the person's story.

Language both forms and informs those participating in the dialogue. It is informative when a person tells their story. The person then says something about themselves, both to us who are listening and to themselves. Language also has the function of shaping us in the sense that we become what we express. If I describe myself as "depressed", it doesn't just express my perception of myself. It also shapes me as a person in relation to others who are part of the dialogue, and it invites others to see me in a similar way. In this way, my person appears identical to my description: "depressed". The formative function of language can be so strong that it "bewitches" (Andersen, 1999). If I and others say enough times that I am "depressed", I will not just be that. Both I and other people may come to believe that "depressed" is something that exists inside me as a characteristic or as a structure. It is an objectification of me as a human being. Language casts a spell on all of us to believe that I am, and will remain, "depressed", and that it is a special trait of mine. By expressing ourselves in this way, we lose the understanding that I can be both "depressed" and "non-depressed" – not either or. My experience of being "depressed" must be talked about in light of the communication and interaction that take place among those present.

"When we say that something 'is', we can come to think that something is like that forever and is not seen in relation to the contexts in which something 'is'". Andersen suggests that we can use "shows itself as" to emphasise that this "something" changes, cannot be fixed and is linked to the context in which "something" shows itself as "something". Passion in a love relationship can show itself differently from the passion someone has in relation to their football team. The second point is that not everything can be expressed linguistically. I can try both to let experiences find their linguistic expression *and, at* the same time, recognise that not everything – perhaps only a small part of my experiences – can be expressed through language.

Andersen (1987, 1995) argues that it could be worrying how professionals, both collectively and individually, have weakened their abilities and opportunities to rely on human experience as a source of knowledge. Perhaps the clearest expression of this is our belief in methods, the need to control conversations and interactions with people, and the demands for efficiency and results understood as what we, as professionals, want to achieve in and with the conversation regardless of participants and context. The more uncertain we become, the greater the need for control and management through established methods of collaboration in various forms of therapy and relief measures. To a lesser extent, we allow ourselves to lose ourselves and our footing and take the transgressive experience seriously. The transgressive experience can help keep us grounded in the situation by showing our uncertainty and, together with others, finding the way forward through dialogue.

Part 1

Professional and historical walks

Chapter 1

Tom Andersen

Lived life, democracy and contexts

This book is a continuation of the one published around 1990, first titled *The Reflective Team* and later *Reflective Processes*. It was translated into nine languages – namely, German, English, American, Hungarian, Danish, Swedish, Spanish, Portuguese and Japanese – and reprinted several times in Scandinavia and South America.

The book described a form of practice that was both simple and powerful, often leading to change in difficult situations. What was new about this form of practice was that everything was done and said in the open. In other words, an audience, albeit a small one, was included. When a witnessing and commenting audience is included, everything that is shown and said is magnified and amplified. Most of the time, this contributed to improvement in difficult situations; sometimes, the situations remained the same, but when the working method was young, we unfortunately also contributed to the worse.

The first book was written within and from a Norwegian context, while this book is written within and from a much larger context. News of this form of dialogue quickly spread to many countries, and invitations soon followed. There have been presentations, practical work, books and articles in more than 50 countries and states across all five continents.

At the same time as the geographical spread, the forms of dialogue have been used in more and more contexts. Before the first book was published, the organisations included: (1) co-operation with employees in the local health and social services in Northern Norway on mental and physical problems, (2) work with psychotic crises, (3) co-operation with physiotherapists in Northern Norway and (4) teaching.

Since the book was published, these have been added: (5) work in a closed prison, (6) large social networks in child and adolescent psychiatry, (7) working with people with congenital or acquired disabilities, (8) research on the process of change, (9) co-operation with leading bureaucrats, (10) mediation to avoid the courtroom, (11) attempts to improve the situation in small areas of the developing world and (12) education in relationships and networking.

Participation in these organisations and communities in different geographical, cultural, political and economic contexts has yielded many and varied experiences. It is the combined experiences from 1 to 12 that this book is based on. The book

DOI: 10.4324/9781003357742-4

is mainly experience-based and only to a small extent "evidence-based", offering "proof" and explanation of what and how it "really" is. The evidence-based part was limited because so little of what I encountered could be explained or proven. Most of it could only be sensed and understood. As a result, the book largely presents not what reality *is*, but what it *can be*, and it doesn't tell you what *to do*, but what you *can* do. The book is therefore *not* a textbook or instruction manual in the traditional sense.

It was the encounters with other people that, first and foremost, provided the important experiences.

Some of them were therapists, some were academics in the humanities, some of them were united in "common idea networks" and some were artists represented by their artworks. Meetings with some of these individuals are discussed. Some were involved in unsuccessful meetings. It has been important to think carefully about these unsuccessful meetings to find out what it is important not to do again. Successful meetings are, of course, encouraging, but it is usually difficult to clarify what contributes to their success. Moreover, when working with people, it's almost impossible to repeat a success. It's better to concentrate on not doing again what you don't *have to* do again.

The open, reflective processes felt better than those led and controlled by "experts". It felt better to create positive descriptions of the people and their lives than to create negative ones. It felt better to let people decide for themselves how to live their lives than to act as an expert telling them what to do. In other words, it was important to avoid being offensive. Where did the interest in such democratic processes come from? Many people are interested in such processes and want to develop them, and for everyone, their interest probably comes from somewhere. For me, it's perhaps connected to something that happened earlier in my life. Perhaps I attach too much importance to history.

A little boy is overwhelmed and challenged

It happened at five o'clock one morning in March 1941. Three men marched into our bedroom. Two were German soldiers with rifles, and the third, who entered the room first, spoke Norwegian. He was wearing a grey windbreaker and a brown bandolier that ran diagonally across his chest and was fastened to a brown belt around his waist, with a pistol holster hanging from the belt. He had blond, wavy hair and told my father to come with them. At that time, the families slept in the same room. My older brother, sister and I watched what was happening from our beds. I was almost five years old, and I sat and watched. My father sat down on the edge of his bed without making a sound, and my mother ran up and down the floor screaming. The words alternated between pleading and cursing, and she cried in anger. My father pulled on his shirt, then long, light grey, home-knitted socks, then his nightie. It was dark grey. His movements were slow and sure. His eyes followed the hands that were working on the clothes, and he didn't look sideways. It seemed like he didn't want to look at us. He put on his grey windbreaker and quietly walked out of the room with the three men behind him, saying in a low voice: "I'll be back soon". We learnt that they had arrested 800 Norwegian teachers, who were initially held at Jørstadmoen (a military camp) for a few weeks before being sent further north by train from Lysaker (a train station close to Oslo). We stood outside the wire fence around the station, my mum, two siblings and I, late one night to catch a glimpse of my father. We stood there with many other people. The teachers came in a row, one by one. Germans with rifles walked on either side of the long line of men. My father passed by without looking sideways. He was silent and looked straight ahead and down, just as when he left the bedroom at home, and he and the others were led into freight cars. I was told that the teachers had been sent to a prison camp on the Russian border, in the very northeast of Norway. A year and a half later, we learnt that they were coming back. We, my mother, my siblings and I turned up at Oslo Central railroad station. But they didn't turn up. The next week we turned up again, and then they came. My father embraced them all, my mother and my siblings, while I stood and watched their joy of reunion, feeling, perhaps for the first time in my life, like an outsider. My father was very different. He had dropsy, they said, and they said it was from malnutrition.

Of course, it was difficult to find words for what had happened. Back then, it wasn't so common to talk and find words; it was more common to hope that everything would be fine by itself. The images stuck, and some words were found: This shouldn't happen! No-one should be exposed to such things! My father never recovered. A year after he became ill, he died. Early one morning, my mother and brother went to the hospital, and I realised it was serious. I went for a walk in the woods and decided to take the most difficult route imaginable, and I was going to do it with skis and poles on. Among other things, I had to climb over and through a fallen spruce tree and climb up a cliff. If I managed to complete the route, my father would survive. When I got home and learnt that he had died, I thought that I hadn't made the route difficult enough. In the spring, during a singing exercise in the choir I sang in, the conductor stopped the choir and said that someone was singing impurely. He divided us into small groups to locate the unclean voice. It was mine. He asked in a very friendly way if I wanted to sing in the alto group, but I said no. I was determined that my singing days were over. It took 30 years before I took up choral singing again.

I have always disliked the terms "treatment" and "therapist(s)". Now, many years later, I think that "taking part in peace work" is a better expression than doing treatment. I think it is peace work that we should be doing, as researchers, clinical practitioners, teachers, colleagues, leaders, public speakers, etc. In order to prepare for and think about my own participation in such peace work, it has been important to follow two guidelines. The first is to endure. At times, when the uphill struggle was long and steep, it could be hard, and at times when I felt like giving up, I called one of three friends who are close to me and said that I couldn't take it anymore. Then, they said, "Hang in there for two more weeks!". I knew they would say that. I guess that's why I called them.

The second guideline can best be expressed as follows: "Get out of the mainstream and go to the margins". Out there, on the fringes, where few people want to be, you get both room to manoeuvre and freedom of thought. In the "mainstream", where "safe" views and opinions are enticed, where you are protected if you only agree with those who are there, and where both prestige and rewards can be offered, thought can easily become unfree. It is better to have the loneliness and coldness of the outer edge than the prison of thoughts. So, what would characterise peace work? I imagine that all perspectives in a situation or "issue" should be able to emerge in discussions about the "situation" or "issue". This means that all voices that want to speak should be heard, and no one should be excluded. In other words, no voice should be prioritised and allowed to dominate, and no voice should be silenced and pushed to the margins.

The fact that the book *Reflective Processes – Conversations and Conversations about Conversations* is being read and its ideas applied in so many contexts in so many countries has been thought-provoking in its own way, especially the fact that it has been so well received in countries that have been subject to totalitarian regimes. This is perhaps based on the book's suggestions: (1) Become a participant rather than an observer. (2) Abandon the idea that people can be changed or controlled from the outside. It is better to co-operate with them in such a way that they themselves find the new possibilities and change from within. (3) Stop discussing and planning in closed rooms. Instead, talk openly with those concerned. (4) Acknowledge the other before this other is recognised. (5) Examine your own practices and thinking and the basic assumptions associated with them.

The world is best served through unity and solidarity. During the short life of this book, we have seen political tendencies moving in the opposite direction. The Western world is shutting itself off from the developing world, which is becoming poorer and poorer. Both market fundamentalism and militant fundamentalism have expanded dramatically throughout the world. Although these two forms of fundamentalism are opposites, what they have in common is that they both promote anarchy. Uncontrolled economic globalisation is growing, and more and more countries are abandoning solidarity in favour of privatising schools and health care. A few years ago, I would have said that technical and economic perspectives had pushed ethical and aesthetic perspectives into the background. Now I'm tempted to say that military and economic perspectives have taken the lead in most fields. So perhaps it's a little naive, in these difficult times, to still believe that openness, questions of co-operation about what and how, listening and being moved by what you hear, sharing time and energy, etc. make any sense at all. Yes, perhaps, and at the same time, it is important to maintain such naivety.

Chapter 2

Historical walks

I, the book's author, perceive this book[1] to be simple and superficial in the sense that it largely adheres to the surface. That is, what you can see, hear, touch, smell and taste, and be moved by. The aim has been to make the text like the oral accounts that audiences in different countries have heard. With their reactions and questions, this collective audience has pushed my thoughts in the direction of what the book is about. The book points out how certain aspects of reality *can be* understood, and how one *can* relate to these aspects of reality. It does not in any way present what reality is, or what one should or should not do in different life situations. In other words, it is not a textbook or instruction manual. It probably emphasises certain elements that are often not emphasised, and vice versa. The book is therefore selective and takes sides.

The reality that meets us, and into which we move, provides opportunities for us to move in more than one way. It suits me to wander, slowly and in constant motion, without stopping. Slow walking feels like the best way to participate. *What* this feels like cannot be described. What makes it feel best cannot be described either. It can only be experienced, and it contributes to all the experiences in life that one is alone in experiencing. Of course, it would have been possible to take long or short runs with rest breaks in between. Then, of course, all the touches would have been different. It would also have been possible to move forward with some kind of machine and sit still and watch. Maybe even be protected from the weather. What kind of touches would occur then?

There are at least two ways to wander. One where the body, with all its senses and expressions, moves about. The feet wander. The gaze wanders. The other is the wandering of the mind. The body can only wander one way at a time, while the mind can wander many ways at the same time, jumping here and there on the roads it has previously travelled. There are many roads to travel. There are those where many not only walk, but walk repeatedly, and there are those that are walked for the first time. No matter what kind of road it is, it will occasionally split. One part may, for example, continue towards the centre, while another part bends towards the periphery: to the outer edges.

Anyone who reaches the point where the road splits in two cannot continue both. What causes you to continue one and not the other? It is easy to think that you are

DOI: 10.4324/9781003357742-5

making a choice, and perhaps you are, if you avoid thinking that it is necessarily a conscious and rational choice. It may be that there is something incomprehensibly attractive about going one way, or something incomprehensibly repulsive about the other that makes it impossible to go there. Sometimes you turn around and go back. It may be common sense that says, for example, "This is downhill, and I had decided to go uphill!". In that case, you have to go back and find the way up. At other times, there may be a creeping discomfort, such as "it feels more and more unsafe", that makes you turn around. And perhaps, as you walk there, your mind wanders to all the roads you've travelled before, separating them into good and bad roads. It can help when you get to the crossroads.

It may be that many people are travelling in herds. When the road divides, it can be good to be many if the choice of road is a matter of common sense. It becomes more difficult if the flock has decided *to* stick together when the path that arouses enthusiasm in some creates inexplicable distaste in others. If you walk alone, you will not encounter such difficulties. The solitary traveller may encounter other difficulties. Perhaps the fear can be great if you take a path that no one has ever travelled before, or the fear can also be great if you leave the path that everyone wanted you to take but failed to do so. How do you deal with these other people's opinions that you've disappointed them or let them down? Fear can become insurmountable if going down a new and uncertain path is followed by the noise of accusations and public condemnation.

It's simply not always easy to find your way on your travels. All parents, children, therapists, teachers, researchers, managers, politicians, etc. have in common that they all move forward along roads that occasionally diverge. Occasionally, someone passes a crossroads and knows for sure where and how to proceed. However, someone may have passed a crossroads without realising it; someone may simply be moving straight ahead. It may be that you are told where to go so that the crossroads' options are never explored. Some people like to be told, while others don't like it but can't help obeying.

The traveller can choose the path, but then the path decides. One walks differently on sharp rocks than on sand. However, the road only requires one way of walking at a time. It can be different if you have to walk the same path with someone else, not least when the other person and you want to proceed differently. There may be so many different wishes that you must opt out of the other person's way. It's similarly difficult when one part of me wants one way and another part of me wants a different and incompatible way. The doubts that arise as a result almost must live on until time shows which way is best. A couple of experiences before the professional period, before school age, left a lasting impression on me, and probably became part of the basis for the journey that took place in my professional life. It started as an intern, then as a general practitioner, then as a psychiatric hospital doctor and finally as a university employee.

As an intern

My first encounter with medical practice as an intern in 1961 was characterised by my experiences and thoughts about participation, openness and collaboration.

The medical education I came from was a crucial starting point. As a new graduate, I was determined to master even the most difficult things. My attitude was also that someone else's problem should be taken over and solved, and that the other person, the patient, should be relieved of the burden. My professional life started in Lillehammer, in the hospital's surgical department. There was a lot to learn and a lot to be overwhelmed by. What left the biggest mark were individual episodes in which two of the surgeons made great impressions. In one case, the chief surgeon approached an elderly woman who came from a remote farm and said:

> You have a gallstone, and it can cause pain, but it's not dangerous to your life. If I were you, I'd probably have it surgically removed. But think about it for a couple of days and then tell us what you prefer.

In another case, a man had fallen from a telephone pole, breaking his back and becoming paralysed below the point of injury. He was already breathing heavily. His wife was there and said they had three small children. The doctor listened carefully as they talked about their family. He said to the man, while also looking at his wife, "We'll take good care of you!" Afterwards, out in the corridor, he said quietly and slowly to the rest of us, "We're not going to do anything. A life on a ventilator is no life for him". It was said with great warmth. What wisdom and courage, I thought.

The "carpenter" in me made me think that orthopaedic surgery would be the future. It could perhaps bring me closer to architecture, which I was so attracted to. In fact, I was so attracted to it during my studies that I had a strong desire, but not enough courage, to drop out of medical school. Perhaps a lack of courage is something you should think more about in your life. Is courage something you have? Or is courage something you get? In other words, perhaps it's better to think about becoming brave rather than being brave. If so, who can you be brave with? Can you choose who? Maybe there is no one. What then?

The surgeons' relationship with time was also impressive. They knew when to wait. They knew exactly when it could no longer be waited for but had to be acted upon. I understood that it was a judgement developed through experience. I thought that I had to let that judgement come into play in my future work. I also encountered the surgeon's sense of time and wholeness in an X-ray doctor. When he showed a picture of a chest where the heart was to be assessed, he said, "I always start looking at what I have *not* been asked to look for. So, in this picture I start with the ribs. Sometimes I actually find something interesting". A great wisdom was expressed as, "When you look straight ahead, remember to pay attention to what you see in the corners of your eyes".

As a general practitioner

This was part of the background when I started as a general practitioner in Northern Norway. I was very surprised at how unprepared I was for a lot of what I was going to be doing. Many of the complaints people came in with were muscle and joint problems, neck, shoulder and back pain and general stiffness and fatigue. I was also unprepared to understand the "sociology" of the disease. There were always many people who were aware of, and interested in, how the sick person was doing. I realised that illness creates a community, and that part of what held this community together was the desire to help, but also fear and helplessness. These experiences gave me a certain urge to understand more of the "sociological". It was extremely thought-provoking that an illness in one person created a network of many interested parties. When there was a visit to the sick person's home, many of the family and neighbours were often gathered in the living room or kitchen. Their often-silent presence conveyed that they were concerned, cared and wanted to do something. It is very easy to misunderstand and believe that such presence is an expression of curiosity. I wanted to understand more about this phenomenon.

As a district doctor, there was no medical or other backup. It was valuable to experience and try to cope with the fear of the unexpected and insurmountable that might come, and to realise that the feeling of being alone increased the fear. I said to myself, "I have to do my best! However, it's the only thing I can do". It made a strong impression how the people in the districts became the best co-operation partners in solving the tasks. They didn't call too late, but fortunately not too early either. They taught me that politeness and friendliness go the furthest.

As I said, I was unprepared for how common joint and muscle problems such as headaches, neck and shoulder pain, back pain, fatigue and stiffness were. They couldn't be talked away, so something had to be done. Men with back pain met in the school's gymnasium, and we tried our best to help loosen up. The exercises that were close to play were the best. The social component was probably not insignificant. When you're bothered and also on sick leave, it's easy to become withdrawn and even marginalised. As a result of these practical experiences, I decided that such bodily ailments would be a main interest in my future as a doctor. But I didn't know how to take it further. The link between me and the patients, namely, the conversations we had together, also obviously became an important topic. We talked about day-to-day life, not least successes, and mostly about that. The warmth that developed in these conversations always stayed with me in other conversations. Conversations, I thought, are such an overarching link in all work that they would become another main interest in my future as a doctor. But how, I didn't know.

As a psychiatric hospital doctor

When I started working as a doctor at Åsgård Hospital in Tromsø, I hoped to find answers to the above questions. That didn't happen, but my encounter with the psychiatric hospital led to completely different and new questions: What can be done to ensure that hospitalisation in Tromsø does not so easily severe the ties between the patient and his or her home environment? It wouldn't take long in a psychiatric hospital before it became difficult to return to family, neighbourhood and workplace. When a person became a patient in a hospital, their ties with family, work and the local community were broken, and it was often impossible to return to where they had come from. Was it possible to find another way of practising psychiatry in which such breaks were not necessary, or, if breaks did occur, could it be made possible for the person to be reunited with their environment and loved ones? Something about the routines felt restrictive, but for a long time, it was impossible to understand what these quite strong feelings were connected to. However, these feelings were convincing enough to look for alternatives. Now, many years later, I think it was the language used in psychiatry that contributed to the unpleasant feelings in question. This language that carried forward and kept the routines going. I'm thinking of the pathology-oriented terms and the use of the verbs *to be* and *to have*. Pathological language most often describes a person's shortcomings, deficiencies and failures, and does not contain formulations to describe successful moments and successes. It contains quite a few categories describing that a person *is* this or that or *has* this or that condition. If the descriptions of what the person *is* or *has* are negative, it can lead to the "patient" and their loved ones seeing limited opportunities in the future.

It was natural to look for an alternative to the inner life of the psychiatric hospital. This meant a way of working that could be practised and applied where the patients belonged. Many people in Troms and Finnmark (the two northernmost counties in Norway) were looking for alternatives. Some of us travelled regularly to selected communities, and in fact, what seemed impossible to solve "inside" could be solved outside. Many different local professionals were involved in this: doctors, social workers, psychologists, public health nurses, physiotherapists, employees at social security offices and social welfare offices. It was important that the local people organised the hours that we worked together. They decided what kinds of tasks we should work on. In principle, they decided how it should be done and whether they should be involved or not. It was important that we saw ourselves as "outsider" assistants who assisted the local professionals as they wanted to be assisted. We should take over as little as possible.

Could a university be a good starting point for finding alternatives? A new form of treatment referred to as family therapy had developed in the United States from an audible and visible business to a worldwide and thriving business. Family therapy is based on the idea that people change with time and context. An important part of a person's context is the relationships with those they are close to, most often the family. To create change is to work with the context. Time is another significant factor. Changes in and of a context need time; otherwise, the context itself will change over time. One of the key aspects of understanding a problem in family therapy is that a problem is closely linked to how you relate to the problem and how you try to solve it. This often happens when you do more of the same. It may be that when a father scolds his teenage son even more, the son becomes even more impossible. After a certain amount of time, the father may get tired and give up scolding, and the son immediately becomes less impossible. While it's obvious and undeniable that context and time are crucial, they often get lost in day-to-day professional deliberations.

As a university employee

At the same time that family therapy was introduced in Norway, it was decided that a university should be established in the city of Tromsø. It could be a starting point where thoughts were given freedom and not tied up in daily routines. I saw this as important. It's only in recent years that I've realised what it's all about, namely, that the language used in a psychiatric institution easily creates strong habits of thought that are difficult to break through and out of.

We first met the field of family therapy in 1973. "We" were about 20 enthusiasts, half from the rural districts of Troms County and half from the city of Tromsø, who met once a month. We practised the new ways of working that we had read about in various key books on family therapy. In addition, we acquired a video player and tried to make our way forward tentatively, fumbling our way ahead. The family therapy field's emphasis on the importance of context and time in people's lives left us wanting more.

At the university, we established a group of seven to work in and with primary health care in Tromsø municipality. The group consisted of three psychiatric nurses, a psychologist and three psychiatrists, and was defined as an independent project. Family doctors were welcome to participate in the treatment sessions, and some did. They had the right to "take the task back" if they were unhappy with what we were doing, but that didn't happen. The close contact meant that those on the front line gradually realised what psychiatry can do something about and what it can't. It was useless to work "psychiatrically" with those who did not perceive their difficulties as "psychiatric". We also took a two-year programme in systems theory-oriented family therapy. The programme brought us into contact with leading professionals both at home and abroad. This provided the impetus for the development of the so-called June seminars, which were organised at various locations in Northern Norway, for the first time in 1983. Some of these gatherings were small, and some were large. From 1988, a similar event was organised in January each year in the city of Tromsø. These gatherings gradually proved to be a meeting place for both professional renewal and reunion, and a community in the North Calotte began to take shape. In 1987, a family therapy programme was started in Northern Norway that also recruited people from Sweden. This community was later continued in a "Development Project on the North Calotte in Systemic Work". In 1988, Finnish colleagues working in Western Lapland joined the programme. They had developed specific network work in connection with psychotic crises (Seikkula & Arnkil, 2013).

Networking

The word "network" has become commonplace. Everyone talks about it, but on closer inspection or reflection, networks are described quite differently. It's common to think of networks as being made up of different relationships, and one relationship is linked to one or more other relationships, making the whole aspect look like a spider's web. A relationship can be said to be a meeting, and it can also be said to be touching. The parties in a relationship *both* touch *and* are touched by each other.

There are different forms of touch, such as a handshake, a pat on the shoulder or a look or words in a conversation. A network is constantly exchanging touches. It is not uncommon to think that the network and the group are shaped by the *inherent powers and characteristics* of the parties. It is perhaps less common to think that the formative power of the network and the group lies in the touches between the parties.

Two different ways of understanding networks persist, and these two ways are linked to two different prejudices.

It is common to think that the network creates the problem – that there is "something wrong with the network" or "something wrong" with the individuals in the network, and that "this wrongness" characterises the network. In this context, the opposite bias is proposed, namely, that it is the problem that creates conversations, and that the conversations create, develop and organise the network. It was Harry Goolishian and Harlene Anderson who came up with this view and presented this idea for the very first time at a seminar we organised in Karasjok. Goolishian said that a problem creates opinions of two kinds: *both* how one can or should understand the problem, *and* how one can or should try to solve it. Conversations evolve around such opinions. In a creative and problem-solving network, one of the things that contributes to such a network is that the members have *reasonably different* opinions *and* can talk to each other about them. Reasonably diverse opinions tend to inspire new opinions and ideas. Moreover, the descriptions that emerge in creative networks are formulated in the language the participants themselves prefer. It is easier to participate in conversations where one's own form of expression is accepted. These were pioneering ways of working, which have in common that they involve open conversations. In parallel with this development, I collaborated with the physiotherapist Gudrun Øvreberg, her teacher Aadel Bülow-Hansen and her younger physiotherapy colleagues. This is discussed later in this book.

This community spread eastwards to Arkhangelsk in Russia, among other things, through an education programme. We emphasised working at their workplaces, with the patients they wanted to work with us on, in their own language. In 1996, Jaakko Seikkula and I launched the idea that groups working in geographically defined areas, and interested in dialogue and networking related to psychotic crises, should form a community of interest. It gathered for the first time in 1996.

The overriding goal is to foster open conversations that minimise the need for heavy psychotropic drugs and admission to psychiatric hospitals. The idea is that the annual meetings will provide an opportunity to exchange experiences on how to organise services, work in individual crises and discuss how to describe this kind of work and the changes it entails. Valuable experience has also been gathered in Uppsala County in Sweden through work with people with congenital or acquired disabilities, as well as in a closed prison in Kalmar, where inmates are given opportunities for open, reflective dialogue.

Note

1 Walks and crossroads.

Part 2

Professional crossroads

Chapter 3

The first experiments and steps

This chapter, which summarises the professional development, starts at the end of the 1960s. My thoughts at the time were that people are driven forward by something that comes from within – by inner psychological forces. It was the psychodynamic theory, ideas inherited from Freud and others, that excited me and inspired my practice. From this period, I particularly remember the counselling sessions in 1972–1973 in Albuquerque, New Mexico, with Heber Hudson, an orthodox psychoanalyst. They were very inspiring. I don't remember him saying anything, but he paid close attention when I read from my notes, and he gave me the opportunity to dwell slowly on the details. These meetings always "lifted" me, and this feeling often lasted several days. What on earth was he doing? One thing seemed clear: his attention was completely focused on *this* conversation and *this* moment – not on anything else. It gave a strong sense that what was being presented was of value. It has been useful for reflection in the years to come. However, while this was going on at the time, there were other things that occupied me more. It was the eagerness for change. The psychodynamic theories were interesting in that they made it possible to explain just about everything, but the practice that followed did not lead to change. The great eagerness for change naturally drew attention to something other than psychodynamics. The ideas from the field of family therapy seemed appealing. Family therapy began "in the shadows" in the USA in the early 1950s, became visible in the 1960s and began to flourish in the 1970s.

There are two concepts that this field emphasises: context and time. People change with time and context, and the most important context is that of those closest to you, namely, your family. This was a good fit for the 20 enthusiasts I mentioned in the previous chapter. We were already oriented towards people's relationships with their local community. There were two main ways of working that we tried initially, and we had now reached 1973/1974. One was called structural therapy, the other strategic. The first is associated with Salvador Minuchin, the second with Jay Haley. These have several similarities. What I am writing now is what *we* thought and did. I'm not at all sure that Haley and Minuchin would have approved of what we did if they had been present. From what we read, we understood that families have certain characteristics that they show in all contexts; as they appear in the therapy sessions, so they *are*. We called this a "pattern". It was believed

DOI: 10.4324/9781003357742-7

that changes in the therapy sessions could also have effects in other contexts. We therefore worked in the *here and now*. As therapists, we had to discover what was missing, find out what was wrong, so to speak, and then suggest what was needed for the family to become more "normal". Of course, in order to define something as "wrong", we had to have ideas about normality, and we used our own ideas about normality as a standard. By working in this way, we turned ourselves into observers, thereby creating distance from those we were observing. Not only that, but we also needed to know what was best for the people we were meeting. That's why we planned the meetings in advance, and we also led them.

In the structural way of working, we tried to focus on the boundaries between the individuals in the family, who was too close and who was too distant in relation to each other? Were the boundaries between adults and children clear and sharp enough? We emphasised what was exchanged between the individuals and, in this way, discovered the power relationships in the family. Who spoke first? Who interrupted whom? Was there someone who always had to have the last word? Was there someone who always submitted and agreed? We were the ones who suggested the things that would bring about change. These were called interventions. We might give them a "homework assignment"; for example, that they should do something different from what they usually did in problematic moments, or that they should do something unexpected or surprising to the others in the family. Alternatively, we might simply redefine the problem so that the negative was suddenly defined as positive and thus lost its (negative) power. Our suggestions were often met with unwillingness and resistance from the families, which could lead to us being even more inventive and coming up with something even more "clever", and being even more persistent in getting the families to accept what we proposed. There was a touch of struggle in this. In fact, I don't think we ever succeeded in changing anyone; in any case, it was rare.

The meeting with Luigi Boscolo and Gianfranco Cecchin from the Milan group was very significant. They wanted to know much *more than* what was happening in the families here and now. They were interested in the extended history of the family, and three generations were often involved in the conversations. They emphasised talking *with* the families, not just *to* them. They were more participants and less observers than we had expected them to be. They used elegant circular questions, emphasised positive descriptions of people's thoughts and actions and avoided negative descriptions. Using circular questions, they asked one person to put themselves in another's perspective. They might ask the son, "What do you think dad thinks about what you just said?" and then follow Dad's reaction with great interest to the son's answer. It's a type of question that brings people closer together, and if phrased in a friendly tone, it does so in a positive way. These questions also help conversations flow more easily. Meeting the Milan group was very liberating. From the end of the 1970s, we increasingly abandoned the structural and strategic approach in favour of the "Milan way". This "way" consists of five phases. In the first phase, the team is alone and formulates a hypothesis, an assumption about how the problem can be understood – based on the prior information they have. For example, it could concern a little boy who has started to act strangely after his grandfather died. The team might think there is a connection between these two events. In the second phase, the team meets the family. It was routine to draw a family map, where at least three generations were visualised, with notes indicating who was close and who was distant. The family, who believe the boy is ill, are asked about the grandfather and his importance in the family. They confirm that he was central and that everyone misses him. Some even wish he could come back. The one who has most reconciled with his absence is the little boy. With their hypothesis confirmed, the team leaves the family to create an intervention in the third phase. In the fourth phase, the team reunites with the family and presents the intervention, which could be:

> We don't think the boy is ill, but very sensitive. By doing the incomprehensible things he does, he's trying to draw everyone's attention away from how much they miss their grandfather. As long as he believes this so strongly in himself, we don't think he can be persuaded to stop doing the peculiar things he does.

Such paradoxical statements, as they were called, easily create both confusion and change. The confusion caused people to stop doing and thinking what they had been doing and thinking. In the fifth phase, the family has gone home, and the team speculates about what will happen to the family. So, the team is with the family in two of the five phases and alone in three.

We tried as hard as we could, and we emphasised good interventions. Typically, we often had difficulty agreeing on what the intervention should be. The person who was supposed to read it out to the family would change it at the last minute to something other than what we had agreed on. Our eagerness for change was great, and so was our imagination. On one occasion, our intervention *was intended to* reach everyone in a family, even someone who was not present. The person who was not present was defined by the family as "the problem". The intervention, which had a friendly content and was kindly worded, was written on a small card and attached to a bouquet of flowers that was sent home to the person not present. We didn't talk about the mixed feelings we all must have had.

Meeting Gregory Bateson and discomfort and doubt

The period 1973–1981 was characterised by eagerness, courage, and great activity. We read Gregory Bateson, including what he said about circularity and linearity. It is linear to imagine that what a person does is caused by a property within the person. Bateson disagreed with this. He said that what one person does can be better understood as a reaction to something that comes from another, and the reaction of one becomes something that the other, in turn, reacts to. This is circular thinking. He even thought that "the mind" was a chain of elements, and that the brain was just one of the many interconnected elements, many of which were outside the person. After that, we, with our methods and interventions, were just one element in the chain through which information flowed. Information was novelty, he said, and novelty is something different from what was there before. When I hear something favourable about a person of whom I previously had negative descriptions, this novelty can change both my perception of him and also my relationship with him. We also read about psychotherapy research, which stated very clearly that relational aspects of psychotherapeutic treatment account for most of the variance when different forms of treatment are compared.

We had grasped all this with our heads. Yet we had so much faith in ourselves that we believed we could create change in other people. We had great faith in the power of our method, not least in the power of our interventions. Why did we think this way? It's not easy to find answers, and in hindsight it's important not to be too critical of oneself. I suppose part of the answer is that it was the zeitgeist. Change was popular. What's more, we were both impressed by and "obedient" to the "big boys" in the field who believed that interventions created change. I must add a small reservation here, because the Milan group itself had some doubts about this: "Can family therapy make change just through our current interview method without necessarily making the final intervention?" (Selvini Palazolli et al., 1980, p. 12).

In the autumn of 1981, our group participated in the Milan group's first international gathering in northern Italy. Around 15 groups from all over the world gathered for two weeks to learn from the Milan group. The gathering, which brought together many experienced and knowledgeable professionals, was overwhelming. Paradoxically, it was after this unprecedented meeting that discomfort began to be felt. It was felt behind the breastbone and tended to rotate. It turned down on the left side, then over to the right, then up, and then back to the left side. One day it was as if the rotating became a voice that asked: "Is this how you want to live your professional life?" The voice probably "meant" that we were on to something "wrong". At first, it was pushed back and ignored with the answer: "We're just doing what we've read and learnt". However, the voice did not calm down and persistently came back with the same question. An outsider who heard the intervention we gave to a family with many difficulties and where one of the difficulties was a very deviant behaviour of an adolescent, said, "The family is being trampled on!" The family was told something to the effect that this young person was "sacrificing" himself for the good of the family. This was a not uncommon formulation from many groups in many countries at the time. When the voice appeared the next time, it got its answer: "No". But what was to be done instead? It was a tough period.

It was tough also because this discomfort and doubt came shortly after our group was dissolved (due to lack of funding) in the autumn of 1981. I had to work with the question: what did we do wrong on that occasion? It was a hard realisation when I understood that we had tried to change the psychiatric system from the outside. The system itself had neither been ready for nor wanted the changes our project represented. We had turned the whole thing upside down. We, the "experts", had "submitted" to the first line and the patients. In mainstream psychiatry, it's the other way around: the patients are at the bottom and the experts at the top, and it's all led from the top. The phenomenon of change was buzzing around unstoppably in my mind. Bateson had hinted at what change was, but what kind of "news" contributes to change?

So, the period 1981–1985 was a time of discomfort and doubt. Shortly after our stay in Italy, we started discussing whether we should stop leaving the families when we made the interventions. What if we stayed in the room and talked loudly while they listened? After all, the people we met were themselves unsure of what to do in and with their lives. Perhaps it could inspire new ideas if they listened to our thoughts? No sooner had the idea been aired than new doubts and uncertainty arose; we might say something that both hurt and offended. Where did the idea that we might hurt come from? Most likely from the conversations we had when the families weren't present, especially when we made the interventions. There, in the closed room, we could easily refer to people as both stubborn and talkative, and perhaps use even more negative words. This fear of hurting kept us from communicating our reactions and our thoughts.

Although we were pretty much oriented towards the interventions, there was a growing interest in the questions in the conversation. We used questions that began with who, what, when, if, how, and which, and we avoided questions that began with *why*. *Why questions* tend to "look for" the reasons why people think the way they do or do what they do. If the recipient of such a question has doubts about whether he is thinking and doing the "right thing", the question can easily lead him to defend what he is thinking and doing instead of letting it go. Instead of *why*, you could perhaps ask, "What contributed?" During our doubts, there were, of course, some things we took with us.

Afterthoughts – Bateson, epistemology and the systemic legacy

> Do not call it hypothesis, even less theory, but the manner of presenting it to the mind.
>
> Georg Christoph Lichtenberg

In all these years, it has been important for me to think about how we think and to try to understand how we understand. This can be called epistemology. Now, though not then, I think of epistemology as the light and shadows of thinking – the transient lights and shadows of thinking. Thinking is an activity, and epistemology is the thinking about this activity. Thinking comes first, then epistemology. At the time, I thought that epistemology was the (transient) scaffolding of thinking. Over the years, there have been some people who were particularly inspiring when we tried to "understand how we understood". Gregory Bateson was one, the "constructivists" were some others, and so were the "social constructionists".

Bateson was important to us from 1974 until 1984, when the "constructivists" came into the picture, and the social constructionists influenced us from late 1988 onwards. I'm not sure what inspires us most right now. Perhaps we have begun to believe in and trust ourselves more, and to make use of our own lights and shadows. Bateson was originally a biologist, and he went to New Guinea to become a social anthropologist. He became a mixture of biologist and social anthropologist. My judgement is that he always remained, first and foremost, a biologist. As both a biologist and a social anthropologist, he always went one level "up" to get a grip on the preconditions or assumptions of thinking, and he encouraged everyone to bring their own assumptions out into the open so that they could study and get to know them. In a somewhat ironic chapter in his book *Mind and Nature* (Bateson, 1979), called "... – every schoolboy knows", he presents some of his assumptions, and I mention some of them here:

Science strengthens or weakens assumptions (hypotheses) but does not prove any. The description and the thing being described are not the same:

- All experience is subjective, and we *create* the image we tend to believe we *are receiving*. The process of creating the image or making meaning goes unnoticed by us, but we become aware of the product, namely, the image or meaning.
- In order to perceive and understand reality, it must be broken down into pieces (make distinctions), but there is not necessarily one (right) way to break it down.
- When a chain composed of equal links is *stretched* (the links are pulled apart), you can predict that it will break, but *you cannot predict in which link.*
- When a moving ball on a table *collides* with a stationary ball (the balls come together), *we can predict where* the latter will roll.
- Language often simplifies and emphasises that "things" have properties. It would be better for descriptions to emphasise that the "thing" is shaped – that it becomes "real" through internal connections and relationships with its surroundings and with the person describing it.
- One's two eyes provide two different versions of the same reality they are looking at. These two versions, when merged into one image, make us see depth – something becomes close, and something becomes distant. What the two eyes see separately becomes a perspective for what the other sees. Similarly, when your two ears hear the same sound slightly differently, you can tell *where* the sound is coming from and turn round to see *what* is coming.

All of the above includes relationships and descriptions of relationships. We also became familiar with other concepts that could describe what happens in relationships:

- Entropy: conditions that are disorganised, unstable, and unpredictable; and negentropy: conditions that are stable, organised, and predictable.
- In linear relationships, something is transferred from one party to another without anything being sent back to the first party. Such linear relationships can be found in the "pleroma", the "non-living world".
- In circular relationships, there is mutual influence between the parties, that is, when one party influences the other, the reaction of the other becomes an

influence back on the first. Such circular relationships are found in "creatures", the "living world".
- We read about logical types, which were supposed to help us understand the "levels" at which different descriptions stood in relation to each other, but it was very difficult to understand.

Bateson was greatly inspired by the Josiah Macy group. It consisted of people from different disciplines: computer science, mathematics, neurophysiology and physics, who together developed ideas about cybernetics and a cybernetic language. What I've summarised above gives you a flavour of it. Cybernetics encompasses ideas about communication and the control of machines and animals. Bateson's definition of "mind" was fascinating: a chain of elements that are interconnected and interact with each other. This means that the person becomes part of "the mind", and that other parties in the chain, the "mind", can be both other people and, not least, nature. The person can influence other parts of this cycle (cycle is my word), but the cycle becomes the context that gives the person both opportunities and limitations for what and how they can influence themselves and those around them. What creates life, or, if you like, creates a flow or communication in the cycle, is the influence from one party that creates something new, that is, something different, in another party. Bateson called such a novelty "an idea". A conversation between people can be an example of such a cycle, as can the connection between the body and the flow of information through various organs. It was in this context that he said that change happens when "a difference makes a difference".

Such circuits, or, in Bateson's words, minds, become recognisable when the flow through the chain follows a certain pattern. For example, the information that flows through the body, both genes and all other parts, causes the body to develop a pattern, with two moving arms and two moving legs, etc. There are some basic "ideas" or some kind of governing "rules" that produce the pattern that connects the parts: "the pattern which connects". This became an important concept for Bateson. As I understand Bateson, such a circuit is linked to other circuits. For example, the cycle through the body is linked to the cycle between members of a society, which in turn is linked to the cycle between a society and nature.

The different patterns are differently changeable. When something in the pleroma ("the non-living world") is thrown out of balance, homeostatic processes occur, that is, an attempt is made to bring everything back to what it was, or at least to an acceptable equilibrium. The importance of the thermostat in maintaining the temperature in a house was used as an example. In creature ("the living world"), however, something that has been thrown out of balance can lead to a new pattern emerging in the cycle. If a new and unfamiliar way of life emerges among some in a society, tensions can be high. If the rules of society fail to produce an acceptable equilibrium between the new and the old, a group within society can break out and create a new society. Bateson called this schizogenesis.

Towards the end of his life, Bateson became increasingly interested in ecological interactions. He firmly believed that the idea that it is possible to exert unilateral influence in such cycles, as mentioned above, is a dangerous one. He saw excessive exploitation of nature as an example of this dangerous idea, with other examples being competition, the exercise of power and, in the worst case, war. For him, words like mutual respect, mutual humility and mutual tolerance became very significant.

Bateson played a major role in our daily work as we spent a lot of time reading and trying to understand him. He helped us with words and expressions to describe what happens between people, so that we had something to "bang the table" with for those who were less concerned with the contextual – those who saw the human condition and human problems as a reflection of something happening inside the person. Bateson pointed out that we relate to others by means of our descriptions of these others. If our descriptions of others are negative, it will easily lead to negative relationships. It was therefore important to seek out as many positive descriptions of others as possible to establish a positive and workable relationship with them. The Milan group was also concerned with positive connotations. Bateson helped provide metaphors and formulations that made it clear to us *what it was important not to do and not to think*. In fact, I think that was the main joy of getting to know Bateson. But I'm not sure how important it was for the daily meetings with the clients. The concept of context was obviously important, and it also helped us to realise that there was always more to a situation than what we saw and heard. We probably became more sensitive to both differences that made differences and differences that didn't make differences. We, or at least I, probably also became more sceptical of the idea that we can change other people "from the outside". A person can only change themselves, and that from within.

The book *Pragmatics of Human Communication* (Watzlawick et al., 1967) proved to be hugely influential in the rapidly growing field of family therapy. Two of the three authors, Paul Watzlawick and Don Jackson, came from the group Bateson worked with. The book describes different power relationships between people and the "command aspect" of communication between them. Jay Haley, who was a third member of Bateson's group, became very interested in power relationships within families. Ironically for Bateson, those closest to him had taken the ideas further in the direction of therapists being able to exert unilateral influence on families. Among other things, this could happen through strategic "tricks". This created a deep rift between Bateson and Haley, but their friendship was not destroyed.

At the beginning of the 1980s, there was a brief and heated debate in the field of family therapy. The discussion centred on the concepts of "homeostasis" and "aesthetics" versus "pragmatics". The "aesthetics" believed that the "pragmatics" wanted therapists to use technical measures to bring families back to a normal equilibrium. The "aesthetes" themselves stood for a more artistic form of therapy that would help families develop something new, moving away from the old equilibrium. Large parts of the field of family therapy were, and many still are, attracted to the idea of describing the family "out there" and "fixing" it using quick, strategic and technical interventions.

Harry Goolishian introduced another biologist to the field of family therapy at a conference in Houston in 1982. It was Humberto Maturana from Chile. This proved to be the start of a reaction against the concepts of structure-, intervention- and solution-oriented therapy, which had now become such big concepts in family therapy. The attention was turned towards the therapists in that the therapists began to turn their attention towards themselves. Whenever Maturana spoke to an audience, he always drew an eye in the top corner of the blackboard to remind us that an observation takes place in the eye of the observer, and the eye "selects" and sees only some of what it can see. The eye makes "distinctions", and the image that emerges is just one of many possible images. He therefore said that we are not talking about "one universe", but rather "multiversa". Not just the eye, but the whole person with the eye is actively involved in the process of creating images. Constructivist and constructivism are terms used to describe this creative process, which was individual in that it took place inside the person creating the images. All this was completely in line with what Bateson had said, but in a way, it made a stronger impression when Maturana presented it in his own way. Perhaps it was his way of presenting, and not primarily what he presented, that made an impression. He often acted like an actor.

Maturana was also concerned with the concepts of structure, structural coupling and perturbation. The latter means something along the lines of intrusion, but directly translated it means disturbance. The verb perturb can be translated as to agitate, disturb, unsettle or bring disturbance. However, no living being can be disturbed beyond its own structural capacity. If it is disturbed beyond what its structure can receive, the being perishes. This is compatible with the book's earlier ideas that it is only suitably unusual influences that create change. A structure can be disrupted by joining it with another structure; for example, two people can be connected through conversation. Autopoiesis was one of the big words introduced by Maturana. It indicates that a human being and its subsystems are self-forming and self-transforming, and thereby self-evolving. A cell can only be, and only develop into, what it has built-in potential for. He used the cell as an example of a subsystem and emphasised the active significance of the cell membrane for what passes in and out of the cell. Instructive interaction can thus become a major problem. Maturana points out that in pleroma you can *discover* an object or phenomenon so that you can *explain what it is* and *predict what might happen to it*, allowing it to be managed and controlled, and such explanations and predictions can be transferred to other contexts at other times. In creatura, you can only *understand* what something *might be in a particular context at a particular time*. Predictions are impossible, and understanding is difficult to generalise.

My meetings with Gudrun Øvreberg, Aadel Bülow-Hansen, Harry Goolishian and John Shotter

The unanswered questions from general practice: "How can we understand, and not least, what can we do about people's musculoskeletal problems?" – had long been waiting for answers. The meetings with the patients in the psychiatric hospital expanded these questions. It turned out that those who had been in the hospital for many years were stiff in their movements and moved with poor balance. They also had a stiff chest and breathed more slowly and less deeply than others. In addition, the muscles in their arms and legs were weak. It was suggested that I talk to Gudrun Øvreberg. With enthusiasm and generosity, she introduced me to a side of reality that was completely new to me. She talked about the interplay between different body movements, and how breathing movements were central to this interplay. Completely free and relaxed breathing leads to breathing movements down through the abdomen all the way to the pelvis, the lower back, the flanks (sides) of the abdomen and back, and in the chest all the way up to the throat. If any of the muscles associated with these areas become tense, the breathing movements will slow down. She also said that pressing your tongue against the back of your teeth, clenching your jaw, or squeezing your eyes tightly, for example, slows down the breathing movements in your stomach. The same thing happens if you clench your hands tightly. She encouraged me to try it on my own body, and I understood the expression "feeling it in your body" better.

There is also a connection the other way round, namely that if you hold your breath, the movements in, for example, the shoulders, pelvis and hips slow down. Gudrun also talked about balance; if you tighten your stomach, your back will be activated and become tight to prevent the tightening of your stomach from pulling your body forwards. The tightening in the abdomen may not be felt, but the pain that follows the tightening in the back is felt. She also said that when muscles have been tensing for a long time, they eventually "give up" and go limp, as I had noticed in the arms and legs of some patients who had been in hospital for a long time. It was like this, she said, that the arms and legs "give up" first, while the central tensions in the stomach, throat and chest last the longest. She also emphasised that people had to stand firmly on the ground. If your knees and hips are tense, you stand unsteadily. She therefore emphasised that ankle, knee and hip mobility had to be practised to improve balance.

Gudrun said something that was as logical as it was astonishing, namely that if you become stiff in the legs and thus have poor balance, you will automatically tighten the muscles in the upper part of the body, in the shoulders and neck, to "help" maintain balance. Therefore, if they managed to let go of the tension and at the same time practise their flexibility and build up the strength in their legs so that they stood upright, the tension and discomfort in their shoulders and neck could disappear on their own. She also said that when the tension was released during the treatment she gave, reactions could occur, sometimes strong and unpleasant reactions in the front of the body, such as palpitations, nausea, dizziness, a feeling of suffocation, anxiety attacks, abdominal bleeding, etc. This meant she had to take a slower approach to resolving the tensions.

Gudrun claimed that it wasn't her massaging hands that released the tension, but that massaging a tense and sore muscle stimulated increased breathing movements that "breathed away" the tension. If you're walking around scared, you can feel the fear as a lump in your stomach. You hold back you're breathing by tightening your stomach in an attempt to keep the fear at bay. Such fear could be linked to an unpredictable and uncomfortable relationship with those you live with.

Meeting Gudrun Øvreberg represented a professional turning point for me. The collaboration we started continued and eventually included several physiotherapists. After Gudrun and I met, emotions such as anxiety, sadness, anger or joy were no longer abstract concepts for something "inside the person". They were linked to the movements of the body, not least the breathing movements. In retrospect, it is difficult to pinpoint out how this expanded view of humanity changed the way I met people. But my attention was different; for example, to the other person's reaction to what I said and did.

Gudrun Øvreberg was asked what should be emphasised in the continuation of her "method". She replied:

> You should go with your instincts. It's intuition that needs to be trained, looking, listening and not least feeling. You must be on the alert all the time for the slightest reaction from the patient. What tells you most about the treatment reaction? Without a doubt, it's respiration (breathing). You can see it and feel it with your hands. The hand that can be opened properly, and is both soft and firm in the grip, can tell you a lot. For example, if I grab the trapezius (the sheath muscle from the shoulder to the neck), I need to have one hand on the thorax (chest). If breathing continues, the trapezius will release and the hand working there will recognise it. It's my fingers and my hands that perceive and tell me what the reactions are. And that's exactly what I mean; the more sensitive our hands become, the more nuanced they can receive the body's responses when we try to stretch our muscles. The more nuanced we feel, the more confident we will be in stopping when we should stop. It is therefore important to develop intuition and the ability to sense. The more we develop these senses, the more difficult tasks we can attempt, because we will know when to stop.

I told her that her sense of context was striking! She replied:

> I think it's because I haven't read and learnt too much. To put it bluntly, I think there's too much emphasis on theory today. They should experience first, then think later. It's my use of the feelings in my hands and my intuition that has led me to where I am today. To avoid repeating mistakes, I think there are certain adjustments that are more demanding than others. Stretching your knees provides a tremendous stimulus to your breathing. By all means, let's not forget to include what so many people misunderstand, namely that in most cases a full stretch of the legs does not just come from working with the legs. The body must also be loosened up before the legs get the full stretch. You must alternate: A little work with the legs, then a little higher in the body, then back to the legs, etc. And finally, the stretch is there, the full stretch, which is a great stimulus for respiration. That's why you must go slowly with your legs. It's so easy to

> go too fast. If you do that, it causes them to defend themselves, and then it can take time for them to fully stretch again. And all that happens with adjustment of respiration too quickly, can also occur with stretching that is done too quickly. If you feel uneasy while stretching your legs, take a break. It's important to let any anxiety regulate how fast you should proceed. If there is a lot of discomfort or anxiety, it may be wise to suggest that he or she should take a break and come back and continue when *the desire* to stretch is there. In other words, when they say they want to stretch and not because we say so. Because that really means that there's something inside them that they're letting go of. When their legs are fully stretched, their breathing can function freely, which is necessary to work with their facial muscles. And not least, be careful about asking. Be discreet and wait. It will come one day by itself.

Gudrun Øvreberg introduced me to Aadel Bülow-Hansen. She had a "being in the world" that made a deep impression. Bülow-Hansen pondered endlessly over new situations she encountered but never took chances. On one occasion, she treated a woman with writer's cramp, and the more the tension was released, the more restless and shakier the woman became. Bülow-Hansen told the doctor who had referred her that she could not continue working because this was outside her experience. Shortly afterwards, she treated another woman who had pain in her neck and shoulders that slowly improved with treatment. But then she got much worse, and "as I sat there prying, I noticed a deep sigh and then she started crying and told me that her father had been captured by the Germans the day before. That's when I realised the connection!"

Bülow-Hansen worked with psychiatrist Trygve Braatøy, who was also interested in the body's muscular tension. He described muscle tension as part of the clamping of affect (emotions), and that this clamping took place together with tension of the jaw, respiratory, and abdominal muscles. He said that muscle tension reflects nervous tension. In the seven years they worked together, they were interested in the function and importance of breathing. Their way of exploring this consisted of him asking her to do this or that in the treatment of patients and then telling him what was happening, or her working on his body and him telling her what was happening. An example of the former was that he asked her to concentrate the massage of a man on the soleus muscle (the flat muscle at the bottom of the calf that runs into the Achilles tendon). When she performed the massage, it was so unexpectedly painful for the man that he kicked her off the bench. When she asked why Braatøy hadn't prepared her, he said that she probably wouldn't have dared to do it. The trust between them passed this test without a hitch. An example of the second was when he lay down on the bench and she worked on his body: We realised the importance of stretching the eye muscles when I did it on him. He was lying down at first and slipped, then his eyes dropped again, and then he said: "That's where respiration comes through it all!" Stretching the eye muscles means that her hands pull the skin around the eyes outwards, and the exhalation, under free conditions, starts as a sea swell at the bottom of the abdomen and moves all the way up to the top of the chest to the throat.

They understood that muscles whose functions are in opposition to each other create balance in the body through mutual and simultaneous opposition. Think of the knee: on the front, you find the muscles that stretch it, and on the back, the muscles that bend it. In the hip, those that stretch are at the back, while those that bend are at the front. When the flexor and extensor muscles in the knee and hip are active at the same time, we can stand and walk in balance. The "flexors" and "extensors" are found in opposition to each other throughout the body, in the knee and hip, but also in the neck, elbow, shoulder and elsewhere. Not least in the face: the flexors "close" the face, the extensors "open" it. When the extensors and flexors are active at the same time, *we are balanced*, and we can walk, stand, and sit as we do. However, there may be situations where the flexors get the upper hand. This can happen when we are scared and try to pull ourselves together, or when we feel sad and want to cry but don't want to do so in the presence of others or are afraid to say something that might hurt others. That's when the benders can "help". If we clench our hands tightly, clench our teeth hard, and cross our arms over our chest and squeeze tightly, fear, crying, and anger are kept at a distance, and words are held back. In such situations, the body tends to close its front and curl up into a foetal position. The "help" provided by the body's flexors can, if it lasts, lead to stiffness, pain and fatigue. Aadel Bülow-Hansen helped people in this situation to stretch, breathe, and release the tension in their muscles.

There were three ways she used to achieve stretching: asking the person to stretch, for example, the knee; stroking the body, for example, the back; or creating a massage grip that caused pain, for example, in the calf. Such a painful grip usually triggers inhalation (inspiration), strangely enough. Breathing in stimulates stretching of the body, which stimulates more breathing in, which stimulates more stretching, which stimulates more breathing in, which stimulates more stretching, etc. When the chest is filled with air and this air is released, some of the tension in the body is also released, including in the legs. It was not the massaging hand on the calf that took away the tension in the calf. The slightly painful massaging of the calf led to more breathing, which in turn "breathed away" the tension and pain in the calf. During this momentum, where the body is stretched, the air is released, and the muscles then relax, the front of the body "opens". If this "opening" is too fast, discomfort can occur at the front of the body, palpitations, nausea, breathlessness, a choking sensation in the throat, a feeling of fainting, etc. In this case, the pace of the treatment must be slowed down so that the whole person can keep up with the change in the body that is taking place. Stretching and releasing can be good for many reasons, namely in situations where the body's internal organs have little freedom of movement; for example, when the chest is so tight that the lungs lose their ability to expand, or when the abdominal wall is tight, the functions inside the stomach, such as the stomach and intestines, can be affected. Or when the pelvic floor is tight, the urinary and genital tracts can be affected. Or when the face is closed and stiff, sinusitis can occur.

I became extremely curious, to say the least. Curious about the unexperienced and unknown that was clearly within myself; curious about insight into a completely different approach to professional influence; curious about Aadel Bülow-Hansen's supreme independence in a different professional understanding, her way of understanding people in the world, her fearless behaviour and complete disregard for her own marketing; curious about what kind of person this was, who had clearly made such a deep impression on so many. At first glance, she was "ordinary", but the moment I felt her working hands, I realised that this was something special. Those hands had to be experienced. It struck me that she had to be a different kind of physiotherapist with such a "hand talent". This talent gave her a different experience from others. Hands and knowledge, curiosity and intuition were talents she possessed in full measure. And courage – courage to follow what she experienced and to stand alone as a physiotherapist. She hardly wrote anything down. She believed that professional practice had to be experienced in one's own body and through one's work with patients. She was not interested in any other form of communication, nor did she seek any kind of mediation. It was always we who sought her out. To put it mildly, she was not always happy about how others practised her physiotherapy. She often said: "They can do what they want, but don't use my name as the basis for their professional practice". Her meeting with Trygve Braatøy was seminal for her further work towards what is now known as psychomotor physiotherapy, a term she did not like. She followed Braatøy's advice never to attend courses or read specialised literature. He probably clearly saw the potential in her self-development, as long as she was not disturbed. Consequently, her professional truth was what she saw and felt. She had no theory that was then transformed into practice. Her professional reality lay in the treatment session and her own reflections on it.

She was clear and professional. It led to a strong sense of closeness. Initially, what I felt in my own body was most different and intense. Gradually, the nuances of insight and reactions emerged. How was I supposed to understand all this? "Use your intuition and imagination!", said Aadel Bülow-Hansen.

> Read the anatomy and feel yourself when you tense up and slow down your breathing and prevent a movement. What does it take to get out of it? If you can feel it in yourself, you can help patients more easily. Try to copy other people's way of moving.

The treatments Aadel Bülow-Hansen gave me can still be felt in my body: her hands, her eyes, her words, her laughter, her enthusiasm, and her irritation. Yes, her entire presence. Many, like me, realised that those firm hands wanted something. When they gripped, her eyes followed closely what was happening. First, a grip in the trapezius (the muscle that runs from the neck to the shoulder). It hurt a little, and she could see a grimace on my face, but she also saw that respiration (breathing) continued. She said, while gripping the trapezius: "If it hurts, just get rid of my hand!" When she got down to my calf and grabbed it, she also saw a grimace, but since she also saw that the breathing continued, she continued to massage, and now she said: "Just keep breathing!" And then, after a few seconds, she laughed and said: "That's it!" What she meant was that the tension in the calf. Then she went back to the trapezius and massaged, laughed again, and said: "Do you feel that it has relaxed there too?" Such moments were magical and made a strong impression. The eyes, the hands, the laughter, and the words worked together and constituted a kind of collective co-movement in my breathing. She became an intense presence that wanted something to happen. Straight to the point. It wasn't about a method, but about human art, namely, following the other person. What was felt in the body during these encounters has stayed with me and has contributed to the development of reflections and ideas about what she did in her interaction with those she treated.

Later, when we made "general observations", such as that she was "suitably unusual" in her relationship with those she treated, neither "too much nor too little unusual", and told her so, she reacted with astonishment: "Am I?" This response led to a new "overarching consideration", namely that her hands quite precisely "knew" what to do, without her mind necessarily grasping it. The hands were constantly assisted by the eyes. The hands and eyes figured out from moment to moment whether what was happening was "suitably unusual" or not. This is an extension, and an important nuance, of what Gregory Bateson wrote about "one difference coming from another difference". When her hand massaged the calf and created a localised change in the muscle, pain arose, which in turn affected and increased breathing, which in turn affected the tension in the calf and "breathed it away". But if something was to happen to the tension in the calf, her hand had to be reasonably active. If it was *too* gentle, nothing happened to the breath; if it was *too* hard or held *too* long, the person took a gasping breath and held it. The person did not let go of the breath. This idea of the "suitably unusual", which I transferred from Aadel Bülow-Hansen's bodywork to psychotherapy, has been a big success in all countries.

When we, as therapists, say something, we need to look carefully at whether the person maintains the desire to participate in the conversation. If the other person is bored, our questions are probably too common. If the other person looks down or away, or doesn't want to join in and talk any more, our questions are probably too unusual; they may have made the other person feel scared, embarrassed, insecure, pained, or sad, etc. There were certainly strong ethical elements in her approach; she was responsible for putting something in place that brought the other person out of a distressing situation, while at the same time she was responsible for ensuring that, in this act of helping, she did not hurt or offend. The unstoppable urge on her part to say: "Don't let me bother you!", "Tell me if it hurts!", "If it's uncomfortable, just get rid of my hand!" is reminiscent of Emmanuel Levinas' philosophy. He said that he preferred to put the philosophy of ethics (here: about the present activity) before the philosophy of ontology (here: about the being of the other). Aadel Bülow-Hansen preferred first to find a relationship with the other (the ethical) before she and the other explored the body's difficulties (the ontological) together. After Levinas had opened one door for another, he said: "Go ahead, I'm coming after you!" ("Aprez vous!"), after which he said: "This is my philosophy". These principles are also important in conversations—namely, to always clarify first *how* we are going to talk to each other *before* we start talking about "the thing". She didn't want to follow any preconceived plan. She drew on an enormous repertoire of experiences that she adapted to the current moment. She would do something, then pay close attention to what it entailed, and proceed on that basis – not on the basis of any preconceived plan. She worked from moment to moment. Her seemingly innocent call to "let your breath go" has always made a strong impression. It has always been like hearing her say "Let go of life!" or "Let life come!" In the echo of that, you can hear: "Don't run after life!" or "You can't control the life that comes! Wait for it to come on its own!" Everyone knows that this is not easy, not least therapists who want to be prepared in advance. It's best to wait until they, the patients, clients or people, or whatever they're called, arrive, and then ask, "How would you like to use this meeting?"

Muscles and breathing – a round-up

Some of the most common tasks for a doctor in general practice were, as previously mentioned, shoulder, neck and back pain, headaches, fatigue, etc. It was not difficult to understand that the muscles in the corresponding areas were tense and painful. In the psychiatric hospital, a new discovery was made – namely that the patients who had been there for many years had flaccid muscles in their legs and arms, and they breathed with great caution. When they had a cold and it was necessary to listen to their chests, it was remarkable that I had to wait a long time for them to breathe, and when they did, their breathing was short and careful. The accumulated interest and the many unanswered questions about the body weighed on me. The meetings with Gudrun Øvreberg and Aadel Bülow-Hansen brought me into a new world, where I am still fully engaged. Aadel Bülow-Hansen became the greatest professional role model for both Gudrun and me. We strongly experienced her "being in the world"; in other words, how she related to reality, not least the people in it. Let me therefore mention a few key points about her working methods.

As everyone knows, our lives are in danger after just a few minutes if we can't breathe. When we breathe in, we take in oxygen, and when we breathe out, we release the body's carbon dioxide. In this vital exchange, the body works steadily through the breathing movements (called respiration in Latin): inhalation (inspiration) and exhalation (expiration). Inhalation occurs when muscles in different parts of the body are active, while exhalation is passive – the air is released. Breathing movements are closely linked to and interact with the body's other muscle movements. The individual muscles have two functions: to create movement and to stop movement. If any of the body's movements stop, this will immediately slow down the breathing movements. For the sake of simplicity, all the body's muscles can be divided into two groups: those that bend (flexors) and those that stretch (extensors). On the back of the knee, we find the flexors, and on the front, the extensors. The "flexors" and "extensors" are opposing forces and are found in opposition throughout the body – as mentioned in the knee, but also in the hip, neck, elbow, shoulder, and not least in the face: the flexors "close" the face, while the extensors "open" it. When the extensors and flexors are active together, *we are balanced*, and we can walk, stand, and sit as we do. However, there may be situations where the flexors gain the upper hand; for example, when we are frightened and try to pull ourselves together, or when we feel sad and want to cry but do not wish to do so in front of others, or when we are afraid to say what is on our minds for fear of hurting someone. Then the flexors can "help". If we clench our hands tightly, grind our teeth, and cross our arms over our chest and squeeze, fear and tears are kept at a distance and words are held back. In such situations, the body tends to close its front and curl up into a foetal position. The "help" provided by the body's flexors can, if it persists, lead to stiffness, pain and fatigue.

Harry from Galveston

The open, reflective conversations were a major event. Another significant event in 1985 was the arrival of Harry (Harold) Goolishian for our June seminar organised that year in Karasjok. I had met him briefly in 1982 and got to know him better in 1984 in Ireland. I thought, "This man is so friendly that he should come to Norway!" He was as important as Aadel Bülow-Hansen, which is why he is also given an important place here, from his first meeting with Norway until his death on 10 November 1991. Harry liked to move along the edge of the unknown, driven by a constant desire to explore where and how one could go further. He disliked the tendency he observed in the field for many to worship the big names and consistently refused countless attempts by others to include him among the "master therapists" or "superstars". It was unthinkable for him to create "The Goolishian School of Therapy", as so many would have wished. What he wanted was to search the horizon of his own thinking to find out what lay beyond what he could already see. In fact, he would have been disappointed if the story about him did not question what he did and thought. What follows, then, is "the story of Harry" as I wish to remember him and as he himself would probably have accepted.

He was quite a bit older than the rest of us and had experienced a great deal, not least adversity. It made a strong impression on me how, in June 1985, he immediately understood my difficult relationship with Norwegian psychiatry. He even recognised my "enemies" long before I had seen them myself. He came as a psychologist to the medical faculty at the University of Texas in Galveston. He was "kindly overlooked" by the rest of the faculty and was therefore given great freedom to experiment. Together with Robert MacGregor and Agnes Ritchie, among others, he developed what later became known as Multiple Impact Therapy (MIT). In this approach, a large team met a family once, for one to three days. If they were to meet again, it happened after several months. This was adapted to long travelling distances and to the fact that the families often had low incomes. During this period, they sought help from Gregory Bateson, long before he was "discovered" by the field. When MIT was at its height, Harry suggested abandoning their established way of working to explore something new. I imagine he said what he often used to say: "Don't fall so much in love with what you're doing that you have to carve it into stone!" Long before MIT, he had already been practising family therapy. A few other therapists in the US had been doing the same thing, without knowing about each other. Meeting not only the identified patient but also other members of the family was a radical break with prevailing practice and thinking, particularly regarding confidentiality and what was considered "good" therapy.

There were big changes in Galveston in the 1970s. New management at the medical faculty constricted Harry and his work, and he and Harlene Anderson started the Galveston Family Institute. This became a Robin Hood institute. Anyone who wanted to could come, and those who had a lot of money paid a lot, while those who had nothing paid nothing. The latter made up the largest part of the client group. Harry was particularly interested in the large and difficult cases that were given up by other practitioners. He called these "chronic treatment failures" and never concealed the fact that we as therapists can contribute to both the better and the worse. That's why he called them treatment errors. Several "psychotics" who had been subjected to "treatment errors" came out of it after meeting Harry. I attended such meetings several times. He also got involved in tasks that are easily defined as social or educational problems. He and others from the institute therefore worked quite extensively with those who belonged to correctional services in the community and those who did not fare well in schools. The institute trained therapists and was a distinctly open institute. Harry installed one-way mirrors everywhere, and no one was allowed to "own" their families. Anyone could follow the ongoing work through one-way mirrors.

Harry always emphasised the importance of having contact with as many people as possible, and at an early stage he became well acquainted with Murray Bowen's work based on the original family, Salvador Minuchin's structural family therapy, Jay Haley's strategic therapy, the Palo Alto Group's interactional therapy, Gregory Bateson's cybernetic thinking, Carl Whitaker's work, and Lynn Hoffman's publications. Harlene Anderson and Paul Dell joined Harry at the medical school. During this period, Harry and Paul regularly travelled to Austin, Texas, to meet and discuss with Ilya Prigogine, who was a chemist. In these discussions, they explored ideas about the relationship between instability in systems and change. Paul and Harry wondered if such considerations could shed light on the changes that take place in families. This happened at a time when the waves in the field of family therapy were running high. On the one hand, there was the homeostasis of families, "bringing them back to what they have always been", and on the other hand, change, "the therapeutic imperative to tear apart the destructive patterns of behaviour in families". Those in favour of the latter were divided into the pragmatic and the aesthetic. It's easy to see how these two words in themselves created strong reactions.

There was a constant search for new perspectives, and Harry became acquainted with Humberto Maturana and his colleague Francisco Varela, who was also a biologist. These two "recurred" in the family therapy field's gatherings over the next 20 years, advocating that our knowledge of others is fundamentally constructed by us, a basic constructivist idea. Harry insisted that there should be a lot of discussion at the institute in Houston. In particular, he challenged prevailing practices and theories, and many of these discussions were open to anyone. Harry primarily sought new metaphors; it was not so important to learn and understand what these different people thought and wrote. He particularly liked what Richard Rorty wrote:

> We see both intellectual and moral progress not as an expression of getting closer to the true or the good or the right, but as an increase in the power of ingenuity. The ability to rewrite the ordinary in unusual terms.

This, I think, is what Harry was doing all the time – unstoppably rewriting the ordinary in unusual ways. Surrounded by people and the questions he liked. Up early the next morning.

Chapter 4

The next experiments and steps

I call it a crossroads because I'm very unsure to what extent this was a choice. It was more like having to give something up – really give it up. We couldn't go on like that any longer; it wasn't working. We had to give it up.

Perseverance – indifference or perseverance?

Two crossroads had already been passed before the professional journey began. In the first, perseverance was separated from indifference. There are certain situations where it is important to do your best to endure and where it is crucial *not to* become indifferent. There are certain values that must be protected and passed on. The values in question probably vary from person to person. What they have in common is that it is in situations where they are threatened with being suppressed that their importance becomes clear. I imagine that everyone has experienced such existential and formative crises. What I encountered is hardly unique in a broad sense, but it was significant, also for my professional life.

The episode from the Second World War when my father was arrested and later died, just after the war, has left a lasting impression. It also burned itself in as a lasting mark. It became important early on that no one should imprison, humiliate, offend, oppress, or separate those who belong together. It is important *not to* become indifferent to values and principles, to obedience and disobedience, and to involuntary poverty and injustice. Something else that happened in the same period was that we children saw others in trouble. There were soldiers being held prisoner by the Germans close to where we lived. We regularly went to the fence around the prison camp and threw food parcels over to the prisoners. When we did this, which was of course illegal, the young German soldiers discreetly turned away and "overlooked" the whole thing. In these encounters between the prisoners, the soldiers, and us, the feeling of solidarity was perhaps awakened for the first time. Something else that was significant at the time was the "Swedish parcels". The Swedes sent small brown cardboard boxes of food for all Norwegian schoolchildren to take home. The chocolate spread was particularly good. The sense of the importance of solidarity was probably further reinforced. In this way, later events remind us of the original experiences and make us relive

DOI: 10.4324/9781003357742-8

them repeatedly. It became important *not to* become indifferent to values and principles, to obedience and disobedience, and not least to justice and injustice. It became important to persevere and protect what had become most valuable. Over the years, it also became important to find out how far the body could endure skiing before it could take no more, or how strong the fear had to become before it was no longer possible to endure it.

The edges – continue in the midstream or head for the edges?

As a general practitioner myself, I had experienced the limited value of sending a patient, with my referral letter, to a specialist and getting the patient back with the specialist's cover letter. This was particularly the case in psychiatry. After returning from the USA, I joined a medical practice in Tromsø and talked to the patients these doctors wanted me to see. During this period, a new crossroads became visible, and a new choice had to be made. It was easy. At this crossroads, you could either continue in the midstream or take the road to the fringes, as I did. The midstream is complex. I have already mentioned that formation takes place. The child imitates and repeats what those around it show and want it to imitate and develop towards. However, there are other imitations and repetitions, namely the fashions of where one goes and how one goes, what one talks about, what one reads and writes, what one is entertained by, and who and what one admires. It is not at all uncommon for it to be difficult to find meaning in such fashions. It's as if fashion takes on a life of its own and sustains the special and exclusive context of which it is a part. I simply became sceptical about midstream fashions. I have been particularly critical of the dominant professional discourse – not just what a dominant party thinks others should be concerned with, but also how one should be concerned with it. The idea of consensus – "agreeing" on one way of understanding and "agreeing" on one way of doing something – can be dangerous when it is possible to both understand and move forward in many ways.

On the fringes, things are freer, and it's possible to apply everything you've been trained to do. Thus, under new circumstances, you repeat what you know in a slightly different way and thereby become a little different yourself. Out there, you can go wherever you want and keep the fashionable at bay. It can come at a cost, namely when fear creeps in; for example, when you get lost and are alone. What's interesting out there is that every now and then you meet others who also favour the outskirts. It's been particularly inspiring to see how they practise their attitudes to life. I met quite a few people like Aadel Bülow-Hansen and Harold Goolishian. The mainstream, the path many follow, is also complex. Part of this current has flowed through generations and shaped those who are affected by it. We need to be part of that flow to be able to pass on values and traditions to those who follow us. Another part consists of transient ways of being – fashions – which we are drawn to in various ways to emulate. It seems that the centre of this part of the midstream is that everyone should be the same: eat the same things, wear the same clothes, talk the same way, be entertained by the same things, laugh at the same things, etc. Be one of a big group. The fear of being different from others draws us back to the herd. Money is power that can be used, especially by those who construct fashions from which to profit, and which draw different people to the herd even if they don't want to be there, feeding their fear of leaving it.

There was never any doubt about following the first part of the midstream. There was never any doubt about leaving the second part because it felt uncomfortable to indulge in ill-founded imitations. One sure way of distancing yourself from the second part of the midstream was to go to the fringes. There, there was more freedom in what you could do and where you could go. The freedom allows you to wander alone, and in various new contexts, to try out on your own what you were formed to be. There is, of course, a danger that being alone too much can lead to loneliness and fear. It turned out that there were some others out there who also wanted to feel their way on their own and develop their education without too much influence from others. Encounters with such fringe people were always inspiring, especially those who quietly went their own way and had no desire to decide, lead, or convince others.

The special and the unusual or the ordinary and the difficult

The third crossroads, which became the first on my professional journey, I encountered on my very first day as a general practitioner in a remote northern district. It was the common and the difficult that captured my interest. The most common was pain in muscles and joints – aches and pains that hampered movement and were aggravated by movement. Such conditions were often part of a life with social difficulties such as poor finances and an uncertain future, or sick children, or a lot of unspoken and unresolved issues between those who lived together. The most difficult situations were those where what was said and done became incomprehensible and unpredictable, creating fear. Such situations could end with hospitalisation in a psychiatric hospital. It was always problematic for both the person who was hospitalised and those who remained at home. Those of us who worked in rural areas had the opportunity to deal with these situations at an early stage. I often felt that I fell short in meeting and doing something about this. Ironically, I wasn't adequately prepared for either the most common or the most difficult. I simply had to start practising and then think. It could have been a choice in favour of the special and unusual. Then the road would probably have led to the central and specialised institutions. That was not attractive. My time in general practice had made me realise that the most common and difficult problems were best dealt with in the local context. That's why I became interested in contexts. That's why it was natural to find forms of practice that *didn't* fragment natural wholes.

Throughout my working life, I have wondered whether programmes for professionals who work with people could start by getting to know practice – what's common and what's unusual in practice, what's difficult and what's trivial. It would be good to learn how to socialise with all kinds of people, both the usual and the unusual, both the difficult and the not so difficult. In this way, the students could learn about the specifics for which they would be trained in the following years – especially for the common and difficult, but of course also for the more particular and rarer.

In medical school, we first learnt about chemical particles and how they bonded to each other. Next, we learnt to recognise the bonds in living things – in blood and body fluids, in cells and various tissues. The next step was to study the various parts of the body, such as bones, muscles, heart, kidneys, and brain, first as dead, later as living. Then, in the middle of the study, we met the whole person, inside the hospitals. Finally, the psychiatric patients. We never met the patients in their homes. As a young, newly qualified doctor, it was in general practice in Northern Norway where I first gained independent professional experience. It forced me to pay attention in almost every direction, and the work I took part in revealed a myriad of future possibilities for a doctor. The rare and special things I encountered could be so unusual that they had to be taken over by those with specialised knowledge in the hospitals. The more special, the more specialised the hospital. My training as a doctor taught me a lot about the special, but I encountered little of it in practice. So, when I did encounter it, those who knew more than I did took over. Pain and stiffness when moving the body were among the most common. Conversations with people were probably the most common, because we had to talk to each other, no matter what the task was. Sometimes these conversations were difficult when new and unfamiliar situations arose and when the usual way of talking wasn't enough. During my education, I had learnt little about the ordinary and difficult things that I now encountered every day.

On some occasions, the most common and ordinary thing, the conversation, also became the most important and difficult. Visiting people's homes when they were ill gave rise to many reflections. Usually, many people were gathered – the sick person's family, and often other relatives and neighbours. The seriousness of their presence was intense and great. Often little was said by the participants, other than that they expressed their desire and readiness to help if desired. The person who was ill was usually in a room inside. I went in and did what I had to do. When I came, I was often able to tell them that it wasn't so bad and that the sick person would be fine. It triggered warmth and joy. Occasionally, when I returned to the kitchen together with the sick person who had returned to normal, the cheers would erupt. The times when I returned to the kitchen and said that this was serious and the patient needed to be hospitalised, both their excitement and desire to help increased. For a long time, I labelled these meetings or gatherings in the kitchens as "the sociology of illness". A case of illness often created a specific and strong commitment in many people. Unanswered questions about how this phenomenon could be understood contributed to my going into psychiatry to find answers. It has been natural to ask how it could be that attention could be drawn to the ordinary and difficult.

Outside – working inside or outside?

As mentioned, the path into psychiatry led to the hope that it could clarify what I have called "the sociology of illness". In connection with home visits, it was easy to realise that the illness of one person involved many people around that person. Both family and neighbours were often present to find out what was wrong and, not least, to help if necessary. Their presence demonstrated compassion and a willingness to participate. It became clear to me that one person's illness could generate such great commitment in many others. At the time, treatment was mainly carried out in psychiatric hospitals. People from Troms and Finnmark counties were sent to Åsgård Hospital in Tromsø. Once there, it didn't take long before it became difficult to reconnect with local communities, work, and even family. It was therefore important to make greater efforts in the local community to prevent the connection from being broken. However, there was something else that contributed to doing this locally, namely, the patients' longing for home and their place of origin. So, a bit of common sense and a good deal of emotion led some of us to make monthly trips out of Tromsø and work in the local communities together with the local professionals. This created several successful results that encouraged us to continue the work "out there". It became a crossroads where my continuation became a prioritisation of the work "outside" over the "inside".

"Inside" only existed in the psychiatric hospitals. Those who had to face it had to leave their homes and go to the hospital. Some came to the hospital because others wanted them to, not because they wanted to themselves. The legislation was such that if "the others" had good reasons, the person could be hospitalised against their will, even by force. It didn't take long for me to realise that those who were admitted in this way lost their connection to where they came from. They also had great difficulty returning home. This immediately led to the idea that we needed to be more "out there" to prevent the connection from being broken. Alongside this viewpoint, there was something else that also contributed to wanting more work "out there". It was how those who weren't allowed to stay at home experienced the unwanted stay "inside". Some of those who came in against their will protested loudly. Most remained silent and said little. We could see that they stood looking out towards the forest, the sea and the mountains, and in their minds, they were probably at home. For those of us who experienced the patients in this way, they were like refugees who had lost their home. Nonetheless, they longed to return to it. We were also used to thinking that the problems the patients "had" or the "deviations" they showed through what they said and did stemmed from "something" inside them. It was our task to "treat" this "something", which we thought followed the person everywhere. We made our attempts to treat, even if we never "discovered" what was wrong.

When we were "out and about", we discovered and experienced that it is natural to think that people behave differently in different contexts. People's behaviour at home became understandable when we saw them in their natural context. Their behaviour became incomprehensible in the artificial context of the hospital. Two elements were central to this way of working: people change with the context in which they live, and the context changes over time. It became natural to go out to the districts and work together with those who were already there and working. So, we left the centre. We realised that it was possible to *avoid* breaking ties with where people belonged. This was far from always successful, but often enough to serve as an encouragement to continue.

Everyday language – expert language or everyday language?

Immediately after the fourth, the fifth fork in the road appeared, and it concerned language. We spoke differently "outside" than "inside". For a long time, there was an inexplicable feeling that it was better to talk the way I did "outside". There, we used everyday language without the expert words. We were naturally interested in what people succeeded with – what enabled them to overcome their difficulties. It was a language that aimed at opportunities and change. "Inside", the language of experts was used. This language was more concerned with faults and shortcomings. The use of pathological language is largely aimed at diagnoses, which easily become static descriptions. It didn't feel right to create static descriptions of people we assumed could change. In other words, it felt better to talk about what people succeeded at rather than what they fell short of. The choice at this crossroads was distinctly emotional. First and foremost, it felt important to get away from the discomfort of being in the pathological language. Since then, it has been important to use *only* everyday language that everyone can understand, both in oral and written professional contexts. If an expert word appears, it must immediately be translated into an everyday expression. This has been an unquestionable requirement for me. Language is an important theme in this book. Since pathological language permeated life in the hospital, it was important to abandon the language habits that existed there. Not abandon them – they were, after all, friends.

A natural consequence of the choices at the fourth and fifth crossroads was to avoid working without the local practitioners. A practical way of achieving this was to avoid having our own rooms. Therefore, when a professional wanted assistance, I travelled to the local helper so that the two of us could work together in her or his room. This has been my way of working over the years. It became more and more common to meet the local helper plus the person seeking help and their loved ones. Gradually, I realised that it was often the case that it was the local helper who wanted to make the referral, while those who "carried" the problem were usually happy with the helper.

It became clear that the relationship between the local helper and the person or persons seeking help was very valuable. One of my tasks became to help protect this relationship. Once I entered such a collaboration as a third party, I was there if they wanted me. However, it has been striking how little I was needed. The most common thing is that a single meeting is sufficient. There were a lot of things that automatically happened "out there", and one thing led to another. The new form of practice, going "out" and working "out there", led to new forms of language and ways of thinking. Out there, it felt most natural to participate in people's own everyday language, not least because it gave us the best opportunity to get on speaking terms with them. We became more and more interested in finding out what people thought and did when they did something that helped them. The successes were given more attention: "How did you do it in the new way?" "What did you think that made you do it in a different and new way?" "Who helped you?" "How did they help you?" and "Will it be of value to take this good experience with you going forward?" Out there, we discovered that the language "inside" was different from the language we were now striving to speak "out". When you get into a speech habit, and everyone around you participates in and maintains the same habit, the first thing you do is join in helplessly: "That's the way it is, and that's the way it should be". Once you're caught up in and participating in a speech habit, it can be difficult to notice it. "Out there", participating in the "language of success", it became clear that we were speaking a completely different language "inside"; a pathological and expert language that described everything people couldn't do or fell short with. It turned out that all the diagnoses that were so central "inside" were actually not necessary in the work "outside". For that reason alone, it felt irrelevant to use them.

It felt best to participate in the everyday language of ordinary people, and the language of experts was abandoned. It felt liberating. This fork in the road was far more significant than I realised at the time. Many years later, it became clear that our expressed words have a formative effect on how we think and act. It has led to many reflections over the years. Why is it so important to pay more attention to the troughs instead of the peaks? It's probably related to the assumption that the "disease" or "wrongdoing" is somewhere inside the person. It comes closer to the surface and can therefore best be described when the person is in the trough. Secondly, there's the assumption that everything that is wrong, unsuccessful and dysfunctional that comes to the surface stems from the "disease" or "wrongness". Then, it is, of course, logical to give these external signs a lot of attention.

But has there been sufficient research into whether these assumptions are valid? Out there, it felt most natural to participate in people's own everyday language, not least because it gave us the best opportunity to get on speaking terms with them. "Out there", we discovered that the language "inside" was different. On the "inside", we hadn't discovered the language we spoke there – and that's human. It probably wasn't the intention of the people "inside" to speak the way that they did. When a person is taken out of their natural context and into a foreign one, those working "inside" will easily forget the natural context. If this happens, it is common to turn attention to "the individual in the patient" and look for explanations for what is wrong inside the person.

"Inside", everyday life was full of routines. Something that made one doubt these routines was that they had not managed to overcome one of psychiatry's major problems: when a person entered psychiatry and became a patient, thereby severing their ties to family, work, and the local community, it was often impossible to return. Was it possible to find another way of practising psychiatry in which such breaks were not necessary, or, if breaks did occur, to enable the person to reunite with their environment and loved ones? At this crossroads, the old road lost its power of attachment. However, there was more that contributed to this. Something about the routines felt restrictive, but for a long time it was impossible to understand what these rather strong feelings were connected to. However, the feelings were convincing enough to look for alternatives. Now, many years later, I think that it was the language used in psychiatry that was in question.

This language, which carried forward and sustained the routines, contributed to the uncomfortable feelings. I'm thinking of the pathology-oriented concepts and the use of the verbs *to be* and *to have*. Pathological language most often describes a person's shortcomings, deficiencies, and failures, and does not contain formulations to describe successful moments and successes. It contains quite a few categories describing that a person *is* this or that or *has* this or that condition. If the descriptions of what the person *is* or *has* are negative, it can lead to the "patient" and their loved ones seeing limited opportunities in the future. The other path has led to a different language, one that emphasises what a person has achieved, a language that describes the circumstances under which this took place, a language that is questioning, for example, whether there are other circumstances that could also lead to a better outcome.

Context and time – the individual perspective or the contextual perspective?

At this crossroads, one path continued in an individual perspective, where what a person says and does reflects the person's inherent characteristics. The other path, which I followed, pointed towards a contextual perspective that was promoted in the field of family therapy. The individual perspective had in many ways fallen short for me. When patients left their domestic circumstances and came to another place, such as a hospital, the difficulties not infrequently lessened. When they returned home, the difficulties often returned. An important part of a person's context is their relationships with those they are close to, such as their family. If you wanted to create change, it was natural to work with the context. Time was another significant factor. Changes in and of a context need time. Time itself changes the context. One of the key aspects of understanding a problem is that a problem is closely linked to how you relate to the problem and how you try to solve it. It often happens that you do more of the same.

This divide became visible and resulted from going "out". The distinction between the individual and the relational or contextual perspective stood out. "Inside", when we forgot the natural context, we looked for explanations within the person. We asked, "Why is it the way it is?" We tried to strengthen all the qualities and abilities we assumed were in there, such as motivation, will, determination, independence, and judgement. "Outside", we investigated what happened in the environment just before the "wrong" thing came to light – not least what happened when the "wrongdoing", after it had become apparent, became less prominent or even disappeared. We often asked, "Who was there when it got better?" and "What did they (the patient and the other person) do when it got better?"

These questions highlighted the importance of family. A family's life changes over time. New family members die or are born. The external environment can change, such as relocation, divorce, or financial and social difficulties. Earlier, in the work at the hospital, patients were removed from their natural context. Attention was focussed on what was inside the person. The "mistake" had to be uncovered, and the changes had to happen inside. "Inside" the hospital, we worked from an individual perspective. This was abandoned when we worked from a contextual or relational (interpersonal) perspective. When working with an individual approach, questions are often asked that start with what, when, where, how, who and why. The question of why is avoided in a relational approach. The word who becomes an important word, combined with others such as what with whom, how with whom, when with whom, or where with whom.

Attention in different human situations can be focussed on three aspects of time: the past, the present, or the future. Questions that relate to this can be "Why did this happen?", "What is this?", or "What should I do?". If the questions towards the past are looking for the causes or *the reason*, it can easily create difficulties, especially if the question is narrowed down to "Who was to blame for this problem?" Conversations around this question can lead to attacks such as "What you did back then is the cause of all the misery", leading to defences: "No, it has nothing to do with this. I was only doing what I was asked to do", which can then be answered with another attack: "Everyone understood that what you did was pointless!", which leads to a defence that takes the form of a counterattack: "Have you completely overlooked what you yourself did? In my opinion, it was much worse than what I did!" Discussions of this nature can easily degenerate into a battle over where to place the blame. That battle can take more energy and cause more discomfort than the original problem. There are often many different factors that contribute to human problems. These are usually interwoven and reinforce each other. Early on, I gave up the idea of *explaining* the cause and then the idea of causes. In the end, I no longer asked questions that begin with *why*. If the people we meet formulate questions with "why", we can rephrase them to: "What could have contributed to this?", which can be taken further to "What could have helped make it all easier?".

Practice comes first, then theory

This fork in the road appeared in academia. It was called path one: "Theory first, then practice", with the subtitle: "Theories determine what practice should be". Mine, and the other path, was called: "Practice first, then theory", with the subtitle: "Practice determines what theories can be". Practice and theory are two aspects of all subjects, but what should the balance between them be? In all forms of practice, there is no doubt: practice comes first, then theories. In academia, there is no doubt either; theory comes first, then practice. Coming first means that it takes most of the attention and energy. I encountered the theories in the books. I met the people in practice. What kind of academic should I become? One in the shadow of the books, or one in the shadow of the people? The answer was self-evident. It had to be practice first and then the theories, even in academia. It was the latter that was difficult because it broke with the expectations there.

In a theory-dominated context, there is an opportunity to gain a broad overview and become a good observer from a distance, learning and recognising the general in the individual. You learn to think clearly and independently. In a practice-dominated context, you must learn to become a participant and get to know what is special about the other person. One learns to feel one's way in collaboration with the other. To succeed, you become dependent on and sensitive to the other person's reaction to what you do and say.

Should people be replaced by books? Books have a big place in academia. It was easy to realise that when I entered. The meetings with books could easily have taken over the meetings with people, and it felt impossible. The Greek verb "theorein" means "to look at". One way of looking is to cast a glance over a field or a phenomenon. You want to see the individual components that are there and how they relate to each other. In other words, you must be able to see them. They must exist as facts. They must exist and be identifiable. The theories you have are both tested and expanded to make them as solid and usable as possible. Theories about humans will therefore include which actual individual elements humans consist of and how these elements relate to each other. The theories say something about what exists "out there" in reality. You take your impressions, which represent descriptions that are brought back to the study chamber to study the relationships. This is how it must necessarily be done. It's hard to understand how it can be done any other way. It is obvious that it is impossible to bring all possible descriptions of reality into the room where they are to be studied. It is only possible to include some of them. Thus, many will have to be left out. And that's the way it must be.

As I said, theories are of great importance in academia. It is important that students learn the theories first, from which practice should be derived. However, difficulties easily arise with this. What about all the things out there that cannot be seen but only sensed? Perhaps sensed as something significant? Everything that is impossible to point to or touch and say: "Look, this is the component I'm talking about!" Reality consists of more elements than the actual. Uncertainty in some practical situations can be an essential element. But what is uncertainty? It's not so easy to point to it or walk over and touch it and say: "Here is uncertainty!"

I took the uncertain path, partly because I had 12 years in practice before university. Strong feelings were also decisive – feelings that perhaps went in the direction of solidarity. One of these feelings was that it was important to take part in ordinary life. In psychiatry, this means first and foremost engaging in ordinary, daily practice. This led to being guided to both the most ordinary and the most important. This ordinariness had to become the framework for, and guide, activities in academia as well. It is also in practice that we get to test whether what we develop leads to the better or the worse. The latter is the most important thing to realise. When dealing with people, especially those who are out of balance and feel inadequate and unsuccessful, it's easy to come up with something that offends and makes the situation even more difficult. Once you have clarified what kind of practices make it worse and what makes it better, it's time for the "theories" – namely, finding out what it is about what we do that leads to the better or the worse. When I entered academia, I wanted to keep in touch with the general challenges of healthcare. It was important not to establish my own private practice. The best way to do this was to avoid having my own rooms. When a professional called and wanted to refer someone, I had to say that unfortunately, since I didn't have a room, I couldn't accept the referral. "I can come to you, and we can meet the task together in your rooms". Since then, this has been the practical way of working; always together with the local helper in their room. This choice, to always work together with the local helper, was conscious and guided by reason. Firstly, because I had a district medical background where I had experienced what it meant to work alone in difficult situations. It can easily invoke fear. Secondly, I've always believed that the already established connection between the local helper and those he or she helps is valuable and should be protected. It is therefore best to attach myself to this local relationship and work within the framework preferred by those in this relationship.

Strong emotions were also crucial to this choice – feelings that favoured solidarity. One of these feelings was that it was important to take part in ordinary life. This would lead to being guided to both the most ordinary and the most important. This ordinary life had to become the framework for and guide the activities in the academic world. It is also in practice that we get to test whether what we develop leads to the better or the worse. The latter is the most important thing to clarify. When dealing with people, especially those who are out of balance and feel inadequate and unsuccessful, it's easy to come up with something that offends and makes the situation even more difficult. Once you have clarified what kind of practices make it worse and what makes it better, it's time for the "theories" – namely, finding out what it is about what we do that makes things better or worse. It wasn't easy to be a hierarchically oriented psychiatrist when working with reflective teams. Talking less and listening more became an important practice at this crossroads in meetings with people.

Change comes from within and cannot be applied from the outside?

In this eighth fork in the road, there was one way forward called "change comes from the outside" and the other called "change comes from the inside". I had long been involved in trying to change from the outside by explaining, persuading, instructing, prescribing, making plans for the other person, guiding, etc. If you think you have the *right* understanding of the situation, it's easy to press on with more persuasion or more structured guidance. If the other person is reluctant to accept and "defends" against influence, this can ironically lead to more influence, which in turn leads to more defence, and so on. In some contexts, this can go a long way. This may apply if unwanted behaviour is to be controlled. That coercion, which may eventually be used, can slowly lead to change, such as obedience. Such a change from the outside leads to a reduction in the other person's repertoire of being. Our tendency to tell families how to live their lives became an uncomfortable burden for me. Naturally enough, this discomfort, a physical discomfort, could only disappear if the idea of changing from the outside was abandoned.

Along the path of "change comes from within", we work with families to find new, unused opportunities to understand and solve problems. Of course, when the new opportunities become available, it must be those who know the problem first-hand who have the right to choose which opportunity they want to use. The choice at this fork in the road was the least rational choice I have ever made. It was driven by a physical discomfort, a sensation.

The connection between the three crossroads probably plays a role in this eighth crossroads. The three emerged around the same time as the eighth. It seems now, when everything can be seen from a distance, that the choices at each of the four crossroads influenced the choices at the others. There was probably some wandering back and forth.

Wait to be invited to both write and speak – don't fight your way through

As previously described, the period in the 1980s was a time of discomfort and doubt. We had discussed whether we should stop leaving the families when we made the interventions. We became concerned about what would happen if we stayed in the room and spoke so that the family listened. The families could be uncertain about what to do in and with their lives. When we talked out loud about our thoughts, it might inspire them to come up with new ideas. Once the idea had been aired, a new doubt and uncertainty arose as to whether we could say something that was both hurtful and offensive. Where did that doubt come from? It probably came from conversations we had without the families present, especially when we were designing interventions. When we were in the closed room, we could refer to and characterise people with negative and derogatory words. The fear of hurting contributed to us not expressing our reactions and our thoughts.

We collaborated with two groups of employees at Åsgård Hospital. One of the groups worked at the outpatient clinic and invited outpatient families. The other group invited hospitalised patients and their families. We worked in the Milan way in both groups. It took place in the basement at Åsgård, where one-way mirrors had been installed between two rooms. After a while, I realised that we were changing the way we delivered the interventions. Until then, we had said: "This is how you should understand it all", and "This is what you should do". The unspoken, what was not said out loud, was: "This is how (we understand) you should understand it all (and not how you understand it yourselves)" and "This (what we ask you to do) is what you should do (and not what you are doing yourselves)". Then we started talking like this: "In addition to what you saw, we have seen this", and "In addition to what you are doing, can you imagine trying this?" It felt better to say it that way, and there was a different atmosphere in the room. There was less tension and less struggle. The leap that took place was to go from an either-or to a both-and attitude. Either-or statements belong to the type of description that explains; this is how it is. Both-and belongs to the type that understands; this is how it can be. This leap, from either/or to both/and, had a big impact on the relationship between them and us. It was also a big leap for the mind, in relation to both clinical and academic work.

Both-and instead of either-or – a big practical and mental leap

At this crossroads, it was impossible to continue along the road I had already travelled for a long time, called either/or. On that road, a statement was either right or wrong, and a description either correct or incorrect – true versus false on that road. When two people make up their minds about what is a right statement or a correct description, they may have different opinions. Not uncommonly, both will think that one is right and the other is wrong, and the discussion becomes about persuading the other to realise that he or she is wrong. Strangely enough, such discussions, which can end in arguments, often take the form of first and foremost asserting that the other is wrong rather than justifying that one is right. It's rarer for the two of them, separately, to think and say, "Maybe we're both wrong?". A life on this either-or path is demanding and easily swings between attacking others and defending oneself. In fact, that's what my colleagues and I did when we were in therapy. If our view of how the problem could be understood differed from the family's, we tried to persuade them to adopt our point of view. When we had different ideas about how to solve the problem, we tried to persuade them. In a sense, we were telling them how to live their lives. At this crossroads, another path emerged, and it was called both-and. On this road, which I took, you're not so much concerned with knowing what's right or wrong, but rather with what's useful or applicable knowledge. Different perceptions do not necessarily have to exclude each other. For example, we started saying to the families we met: "… in addition to what you have understood about the situation you are facing, we have understood this…", or: "… in addition to what you have tried to do, maybe you could also try this…". On this both-and path, there was immediately less of the tension and conflict in relation to the families that was so common on the either-or path. However, a paradox emerges here: how is it possible to hold on to *both*-and and either-or?

Speaking in the open – shaping us in other ways

At this fork in the road, one path continued, called "conversations in the closed rooms", while another was called "open dialogue". From the mid-1970s, it was common for us in the team to talk to families about what *we* thought it was important to talk about. After we had received sufficient information, the meeting would take a break, and the family and the team would go to separate rooms. In our closed room, the team's closed room, we deduced what should be said to the family. We drew up an intervention and an understanding of the problem, as well as a proposal for solving it. This intervention was read aloud to the family after we reunited with them. The change came when we thought we could ask the family if it might be of value for them to see and hear how we eased our way to the alternative possibilities. We questioned what might happen if we stopped going to another, closed room and instead talked together in the presence and hearing of the family. Immediately, we pushed the thought away. We were worried that we might speak negatively and hurtfully about the family. This fear had its origins in how we might talk about the families when we were without them in the closed rooms.

The first time we tried out our new way of working, the experience was overwhelming. It was entirely possible to avoid hurtful speech. It wasn't long before we realised that speaking politely comes naturally when talking in public. We didn't immediately realise what felt so good about this new way of working. Our understanding of what this new way of working encompasses has been steadily developed, and our understanding will probably continue to grow and expand. It was the relief of having entered the open road that was so liberating. The open road is well within the road called practice first, then theory, with the subtitle practice determines the theories.

From the outset, we avoided creating one form of reflective conversation(s). There had to be an openness to diversity, and these conversations could take different forms. Sometimes the reflections consisted of soliloquies from individuals. Sometimes they were conversations among themselves, sometimes they were highly intellectual, and sometimes they were highly emotional. It wasn't long before we stopped turning the sound and light round and switched rooms instead. The family and the person talking to them went behind the mirror and the team in front. It felt more natural for the reflective team to put themselves in the family's place when they talked. We became more equal. At first, it felt a bit strange when we passed each other at the door. We didn't really know where to look. Gradually, it became more normal. We were able to smile at each other and say a few nice words. And it didn't take long before it could all be done without one-way mirrors. The team then sat back in the room and listened to the conversation between the family and the therapist, after which they gave their reactions from the same slightly withdrawn position. We suddenly had many practical options. The last one, doing everything in the same room, made it possible to conduct such conversations in people's homes. The size of the team has also subsequently proved to be able to vary from working alone to over a hundred people. My personal favourite is a team of two.

From the very beginning of this new endeavour, we always told families when they first arrived that they had an opportunity to meet and work with a team. The therapist always met with the family alone during this orientation, and the team sat and waited elsewhere. The families got to see the rooms and the one-way mirror. They got to know how it all worked and what the thoughts behind it were: "several see more than one" and "several think more than one". We made no secret of the fact that we thought this was a good way of working. Of course, if they didn't want this form, the therapist talked to them alone. If they were in doubt, the therapist said that they could talk alone before deciding. *Initially*, in perhaps both the first and second year after we started, we probably still had the desire to change. Even though we were sitting in another room, we were probably talking *to* them. At least I was aware that there were recipients for what I was saying.

Initially, it was difficult to understand what was happening in this new process. The first description was that this contributed to a shift from a hierarchical to a heterarchical relationship. Most people understand the word hierarchical without further ado. Far from everyone knows the word heterarchical. That was interesting. Both words contain the Greek verb archein, meaning "to rule" or "to govern". Hieros translates as "from above" or "from the gods", and heteros as "through the other". In other words, we used to govern everything from above, but in the new system, everything was governed through the other — that is, through the community.

We want them to tell us what we want to hear or to let them tell us what they want us to hear – hear what they really say, not what they really mean

It was as if the open road quickly led to new forms of practice. One of the two paths in this new divide was called "let them tell us what they want us to hear", while the other was called "we want them to tell us what we want to hear". It was now only possible to proceed along the first of these two paths. In a way, there was no question of a choice. Rather, it was a profound way of being – a way of participating in the company of others. Nonetheless, it has been one of the most demanding choices. The demanding thing was to give up and abandon the other of these two paths. We had to give up making and following plans for the conversations. Working towards a fixed, specific goal had to be given up. The idea of being a leader had to be abandoned. The idea that it is first and foremost important to solve a problem had to be given up. It was about giving up an entire practice. It was about giving up a way of being in the world as a professional. What would it take to manage and give this up, as long as the ideals, requirements and expectations that a university teacher, for example, must live up to are to lead others to something specific, or be the one who clarifies, or the one who points out the right thing, or be the good model to be emulated, etc.? The walks were probably characterised by walking in circles. In fact, it took quite a lot of courage to continue on the path on which it was simultaneously inevitable to continue. And it took some time to be able to continue wholeheartedly on this path. It took a long time to realise what was so crucially important at this crossroads. The choice felt both right and hard to make.

New important questions now emerged, for example: Who wants to speak and who wants to remain silent? It has become important that anyone in a meeting who does not want to speak should be allowed to do so. Also, those who want to speak – what do they want to talk about? It's important that they're not allowed to talk about what they don't want to talk about. Who is prepared to talk to whom, about what topic, in what way and at what time? Is what is being talked about unusual enough (suitably unusual) to make it engaging and stimulating to talk about? Or is it so like the usual way of talking that it becomes boring and the engagement disappears? Or is it so unusual that it becomes uncomfortable and perhaps even so frightening that you lose the desire to talk?

Observation or participation?

It now became clear that a new junction had been crossed. One path was called "observation" and the other was called "participation". The journey continued along the one called "participation". It's interesting that it hasn't been easy to establish where and when this fork in the road was crossed. It must have been during a myriad of crossroads, and the continuation must have been self-evident. It became participation because the other path, being an observer, felt like a failure. The extreme observer function of studying and describing the other from a distance, from the observer's perspective alone, had already been abandoned. The monological conversations that follow such observer functions, namely that the observer is there to ask and the other person is only there to answer, were also abandoned. Monological conversations consist of many short, consecutive exchanges such as: Conversation 1: Are you okay? Answer. Conversation 2: (a) Are you sleeping well? No. (b) Is it difficult to fall asleep, or do you wake up early? I wake up early. Conversation 3: Do you have many friends? Yes.

There is something else above that also needs to be nuanced. There are situations where most of us would prefer a capable observer who is good at leading monological conversations; for example, in the event of an accident where the injuries to the body are extensive and incalculable. In situations where it is important to find explanations for what is happening and to be able to predict what might happen, it is good to have someone there who knows the necessary questions, especially if time is short. However, there are other situations where you can't explain what's happening, but you can understand what it might be and realise that it might be different under different circumstances. There are even situations where you can neither explain nor understand, but where you can only sense how to act. In the last two situations, it may be appropriate to use the dialogical form of conversation, where we jointly seek out the next step.

As a participant, you become engaged in dialogical conversations, which are characterised by the fact that all participants can both ask and answer, and everyone does this from their own perspective. Everyone is "in", and everyone is responsible for how they participate. To varying degrees, participants allow themselves to be touched and carried away by the others' expressions and give back what the others' expressions do to them. It's important to give something back. Harry Goolishian used to say that an answer requires a (new) question, that is, the answer creates the question and not the other way round. In this form of conversation, we, the professionals, become like an audience that meets, witnesses and is touched by the other person's expression, and we give back what the other person's expression did to us. In this form of dialogue, listening becomes far more important than expressing ourselves. If you think of expressing yourself as asserting yourself, listening becomes more important than asserting yourself. What we give back is often a question. Our opinions and standpoints are less important because they always come from our perspective and not the other person's. What's more, the people we meet usually already have enough opinions. However, this last point needs to be nuanced because sometimes there are too many questions and not enough opinions, such as when a manager in a hierarchical treatment centre, in a misunderstood democratic spirit, never finishes asking his subordinates what they think, instead of summarising when he has heard enough that this is what he thinks they should do.

Ontology first or ethics first?

A central part of conversation, interaction, and togetherness, both in practical work and research, is working with the questions "What is this?" and "How should one relate to this?". I would call the first question an ontological question and the second an ethical question. By ontological, I mean that the question seeks a description of *its* (the being's) essence. By ethical, I mean that the question is searching for a way of acting on *it*, which is an ethical act — at least when *it* concerns a human being. Both questions are relevant in both practice and research. At the same time, a new question arises: does the work on one question affect the work on the other? If so, which question should be prioritised and worked on first and foremost?

Let's take the example of a silent man looking around uneasily. He seemed to be looking for something. Others around him didn't look around like that, so he stood out. His mother called for help to understand what this was. The therapist who arrived first enquired what the man thought about his mother's enquiry. It became clear that he, who had now become even more agitated, would never have called a therapist if his mother had not done so. That's why the therapist suggested that they talk further with the mother. He immediately calmed down, but his mother didn't like this approach and called in another therapist. The other therapist, a well-liked person, brought with him several ready-made questions that he often used in such situations. The man, who again became agitated, was asked: "Do you hear voices?" He became even more agitated and said, "No". The therapist thought that the man's agitation was an indication that he was actually hearing voices, but the therapist kept this to himself. The man was hearing voices, and had been for quite some time, but he had kept it to himself. He had a friend who had been in the same situation and who told a therapist that he was hearing voices. As a result, the therapist and his family demanded that he be treated because they thought it was in his best interests. However, this treatment was of such a nature that it ended in war between the man and those who wanted to change him. The first therapist prioritised the ethical question and left the ontological question to wait. The second prioritised the ontological, and the ethical act, the examination, was characterised by this prioritisation. When this crossroads was passed, where one path was called "ontology first, then ethics", and the other "ethics first, then ontology", it became clear that I had already been on the latter path for a while – probably quite a while. It wasn't easy to work out where and when this fork in the road was crossed. This has probably had a lot to do with the fact that research questions were raised, especially when they were of an ontological nature and were claimed to be innocent.

Human beings are assumed to be permanent – or are they constantly moving and changing?

For a long time, I've walked the path of "practice first, then theory". This means that research must place itself at the service of practice. Research and practice have both commonalities and differences. Both are endeavours in search of knowledge. The practitioner searches for knowledge that can contribute to work that is local in time and place. Knowledge is correspondingly localised. Research seeks knowledge that can help in more than one situation; in other words, knowledge that can be applied in several different places and at several different times. Knowledge thus becomes general. It is different types of general knowledge that the practitioner can benefit from, such as the ontological question: "What is the human thing that is relevant to practice (what is the other)?"

Most, probably all, would agree that in the human (in the other) there is a biological side, as well as a personal, conscious, and emotional side, and a social side. A discussion that has been going on for two and a half thousand years has searched for an answer to the extent to which humans are unchangeable or changeable. Parmenides believed that they are unchangeable and Heraclitus that they are changeable. Today, some believe that unchanging genes and stable brain structures have a major impact on a person's life. Some assume that stable psychological structures "decide" what you think and say. Some assume that stable social structures give people social roles and social functions. Others, those who think that the human tendency to change is greater and that it is bound by stable repetitions, have other assumptions. On the biological side, they emphasise that breathing, which is constantly changing, and the body's movements, which are constantly changing, have a major impact on what a person says and does. On the personal, conscious, and emotional side, they emphasise the great influence a person's inner and outer voices have on what they do and think. On the social side, they point out that individuals participate in their relationships with other people in different ways. In these ties, the person connects to others with both their expressions and impressions. One person's expressions, for example, speech, gaze and touch, are filled with meaning and become the other person's impressions. These impressions move the other to a reaction, for example, a thought or a feeling, and that reaction is given back to the other.

Here we see a crossroads where one path was called "human is assumed to be permanent" and the other was called "human is constantly moving and changing". The choice of which path to take has been built up over a long period of time, and it has been well thought out. It has been built on all the experiences that have been gathered over many years about those who have been stuck for a long time, and who have moved and changed. The interesting thing is that many of those who were stuck and seemed unchangeable did so under certain conditions. This happened, for example, when others wanted to change them in a direction they themselves did not want. When they were allowed to decide for themselves, both what, when and how, the changes came, both in their breathing and movements and in their inner and outer conversations. On this path, the assumption has been made that the human being is first and foremost a participant in bonds with others. However, humans can only participate with the voices and movements they have.

My description of reality is my reality

The world we live in demands our participation. Whether we are doctors or patients, mothers or fathers, drivers or teachers, cooks or comforters, we all demand attention. After all, most of us are all these things and more in a day. Life touches us from moment to moment and demands that we relate to it. We do, whether we want to or not.

When we relate to what surrounds us, reality, we do so with the help of our descriptions of this reality. Many people think that we have direct access to reality and that we can create descriptions that copy and represent it. This is one assumption. Perhaps it happens in some cases; for example, when a door slams and hits you on the head. But this rarely happens. As a rule, we are connected to reality through our descriptions of it. In other words, this is a different type of assumption from the first. Strangely enough, based on this last assumption, our descriptions have double and opposite functions: they both connect us to and keep us separate from reality.

Secondly, I think that reality is complex and basically consists of three different parts, and that there are several types of descriptions that each fit the three parts of reality. One part of reality can be perceived, and it stands still like the Norwegian mountain Tromsdalstind. It stands there, winter and summer, in sun and rain. We can see it and enjoy its splendour. We can walk on it and lie down on it and smell the wet earth between the stones. We can measure its volume; we can take small pieces of it here and there, from both the exterior and the interior, crush the pieces and analyse their composition and finally say: "This is Tromsdalstind. It's so and so big, it weighs so and so much, and there's so and so much lime in it and so and so much phosphate", etc. When you can hit the table with so many facts, many a doubter can be silenced. What's more, those in the know can tell you what would happen if you dropped such and such a big bomb on it. All this knowledge about Tromsdalstind can also be used in other contexts; for example, when assessing other mountains around Tromsø, and it can be used at another time, for example in a hundred years. Such knowledge is reproduced in descriptions that explain and predict and are generally applicable.

Another part of reality is moving – such as a human being. One of them, the one in the yellow tracksuit, says: "Look, there's a man walking over there on the back of Tromsdalstind. A few minutes ago he looked blue, but now he certainly looks red!" "Yes", says the other man in the green tracksuit, "he took off his blue windcheater a little while ago". "Oh, yes", says the first, "he probably got sweaty on the hard climb". The knowledge about this man must be formulated using different descriptions than those that could be used about Tromsdalstind. The descriptions say that he is there, but that he changes with time and context. In such descriptions, it is better to use words like "I understand what it could be". This implicitly says that I realise that at another time and in another context it could be different. For example, if the terrain had been flat and it had been colder, the man might have looked blue all the time. The man himself noticed that he occasionally had to stop and smile because of the beautiful view, and he also noticed that he continued to walk smiling. At one point, when the light suddenly changed, as so often happens here in the north, the view suddenly became unbearably beautiful, and he was horrified that he felt like crying. That's how beautiful it was. He continued slowly onwards, wondering what it was that gripped him so strongly. He didn't understand it, but he realised that he was now walking differently than before, a little reverently, in a way. He had felt something in his body. In such situations, it is perhaps understanding rather than description that takes us forward. The descriptions that perhaps best fit such occasions are along the lines of: I sense that there is something here, but I don't know what it is. However, I sense how I should relate to it. Reality, which is thus complex and requires our participation, thus indirectly requires us to be able to create descriptions at all three levels, namely, those that explain, those that understand and those that sense.

However, as a reader of descriptions, academic and otherwise, I am often struck by the fact that the descriptions and what is described do not match. Some descriptions may come to explain where one should have said that this is how it can be. You might be tempted to say that the blue man is sensitive, and during periods of crying you might even say that he's depressed. If you describe him in this way, how will it affect your relationship with him? What would the relationship be like if you instead said: "He certainly swings with nature, soon he's smiling with joy and soon he's crying with overwhelm!" Yes, descriptions are stories – very often different stories about the same thing. Even if the stories about the same thing are different, they all have in common that they are simplifications. Firstly, these stories arise as a sensed story, then they are simplified into an imagined story, then simplified into a spoken story, and then simplified further into a written story. Despite all the simplifications, we need them to connect us to reality. We often find ourselves in situations that require stories with all three descriptions.

However, it is my assumption that it is with the help of descriptions of the types "I understand what it can be" and "I sense how to act" that we particularly need to move forward. It is far less often that we need descriptions of the type "this is how it is".

As both practitioners and researchers, we are constantly trying to recognise the possibilities and limitations of the reality we participate in. The practitioner often has a localised view of what is happening now in a particular place, while the researcher looks beyond the present and the local place.

When I re-read what has been written so far about the crossroads, it is striking how important it has been to see. It was important to notice the crossroads that appeared, not least to see the new roads taking off. It was as if the sense of sight was given priority over the other senses. And of course, that's not possible. After all, there were many other things happening on these journeys, not least those that could be heard. Heard and seen, that is. If I looked a little to the sides, and not least looked backwards, it was noticeable that some of the walks were walked alone, but far from all. Sometimes they were walked with one other person, sometimes with several. Some of these I continued walking with, while others were left behind. It was far from random who I continued with and who I left behind. It depended quite closely on what they told me and what they were willing to hear, for example, when a fork in the road appeared and the journey should continue this way and not the other.

It can be hard to walk away from the conversations you've started with someone else, but sometimes it's necessary, especially if you are drawn into a form of conversation that steers your speech and thoughts in directions that feel uncomfortable. This could, for example, involve conversations in which many strong points of view are taken: "That's what you should do!", "That's absolutely not what you should do!", "You can't think like that!", "That's not what people who really know what they're doing do!", "The majority thinks this way, so you should do the same!" Or those conversations where others are easily categorised: "She's strong", "He's cranky", "She's always on the defensive", "He's unreliable", "She's clever and knows how to get her way", "He's dishonest". Before abandoning such conversations, it might be a good idea to test the waters: "Is he fidgety all the time, or does it come and go?", "What makes him more fidgety?", "Is he fidgety, or does he get fidgety?" If the answer "He's fidgety" is repeated, without opening the door to any other puzzlement, it may be wise to stop participating in the conversation – to protect yourself from the speech and thinking you don't want to get into. What about those you continue to walk with? They tend to see something not only from their own perspective but also from someone else's. One man wanted to climb a snow mountain that was steep at the sides but flat as a roof at the top. During the ascent, an eagle came sailing by. He developed a relationship with the eagle, in addition to the relationship he had with the mountain. The eagle disappeared but came back, again and again. It had obviously also developed a relationship with him. He began to see the mountain and himself through the eagle's eyes, at the same time as he saw the eagle and the mountain through his own eyes. Participation in a conversation is a way of *being in the world*. It's important to clarify who you want to be in the world with.

Chapter 5

About reflective teams and processes

As written earlier, in the autumn of 1984, I noticed that we changed the way we "delivered" the interventions. We were now two groups. Each of the groups met half a day a week in two rooms with one-way mirrors in the basement of Åsgård Psychiatric Hospital. Since then, I've often thought of this as a "basement activity". Until this autumn, we had said, "This is how you should understand it all", and "This is what you should do". The unspoken, what was not said out loud, was: "This is how we understand everything, not how you understand it", and "This is what we are asking you to do, not what you are doing". In the autumn of 1984, we started talking like this: "In addition to what you saw, we've seen this", and "In addition to what you're doing, can you imagine trying this?" It felt better to say it that way, and there was a different atmosphere in the room. There was less tension and less conflict.

The leap that took place here was to move from an either-or to a both-and attitude. Either-or statements belong to the type of description that explains; that's how it is, while both-and belongs to the type that understands; that's how it can be. This leap, from either/or to both/and, had a big impact on the relationship between them and us. It was also a big leap for the mind, both in relation to clinical work and in relation to academic work. Then, one day in March 1985, we dared to talk in the open. It happened during a period that was quite dramatic for Åsgård Hospital. There were major difficulties on the wards, including a lack of nurses to run the day-to-day operations. The difficulties were also defined as a lack of specialists in psychiatry. There were major headlines in the country's newspapers with many mentions of how short we had come up here. Among other things, some professionals pointed out how much northern Norway lacked compared to what existed in the south of the country. An air bridge was set up, where psychiatric nurses and psychiatrists were flown in to work for two-week periods. It was a tough period for many people.

On a Thursday afternoon, during all this turmoil, one group met to talk to a family of three. A woman in her mid-fifties had been depressed and unhappy for several years, and she had thought about and even attempted suicide. There had been several stays at Åsgård, also against her will. We met her, her husband and her daughter. All three were despondent, and all found it difficult to see a hopeful

DOI: 10.4324/9781003357742-9

future, carrying a pessimistic mood in the interview room. We asked the colleague, who was talking to them, to come to our room and suggested a couple of optimistic questions for him. But shortly after the questions were given, they were all back in the pessimistic mood. We asked the colleague to come out twice more, but each time the same sequence persisted, back to the pessimistic. That's when the idea of talking in the open emerged. What's more, the rooms were double-equipped; both speakers and microphones were in each room, something we hadn't noticed before. We had a brief discussion in our room, and the three of us agreed to give it a try. It was my job to knock on the door of the others' room and say something like this: "Would you like to hear what we're thinking?" Nervous as I was, I hoped they would say no. But no, they wanted to hear. The colleague was unsure and surprised when I said he could stay with the family while we talked. This was a break from the Milan way, where the interviewer in such situations left the family and joined the team. We used the double equipment so that the lights were switched off and the speakers switched on in their room. The opposite happened with us: the lights came on and the speakers switched off. It's still easy to relive the clicks of the neon lights when they came on in our room. For a moment, it almost felt like sitting "undressed", and it was natural to think: "This is how families have always felt; now we can experience a bit of the same". We started off hesitantly and cautiously, suggesting that perhaps the situation was so difficult that it wasn't easy to find new opportunities. Slowly, we continued to wonder what kind of opportunities there might be, and our discussion became more and more lively as we thought about this and that possibility. By the time we turned on the lights and sound, the atmosphere in the other room was livelier, and the three members of the family had started talking about what they could do during the upcoming Easter holidays. Not only that, but they were also looking further into the future and discussing what they could do after Easter. For myself, I thought: "This is something completely new! I've never done anything like this before! I want to do this from now on, because this is a great relief!" Yes, I was talking to myself with exclamation marks. The name of it all also came immediately: "Reflective Team".

Sure enough, the next Thursday morning, the other group worked in the same way, and the group above repeated it in the afternoon. It almost came as a shock to realise that it was so easy to talk without coming close to hurtful words and expressions. It certainly gave me a lot of food for thought, and I gradually realised that the way we talk is, of course, affected by the context of the conversation. It was in the closed rooms, where we were alone without an audience, that it was easy to speak "rudely". Now, in the open, with the people we were talking about as listeners, it was natural to speak "politely".

Another "spontaneous" change that gradually became noticeable was that the group behind the mirror increasingly followed the family conversations in silence. Previously, while we were working in the Milan way, those behind the mirror used to engage in lively discussions to arrive at a common view and prepare a joint intervention. From now on, all the listeners gathered around their own impressions and reactions. They expressed themselves when they reflected on the family conversation. This meant that each member of the reflective group could present their own picture of the situation.

Another description was that this way of working could be seen as a shift back and forth between outer and inner conversations. One participant switched between talking about certain topics in the open, external conversations and then sitting back, listening to others talk about this conversation and thinking about (talking to yourself in an internal conversation about) what you hear. It didn't take long after that description for me to realise that this is something fundamentally human: namely, in one moment talking to others and in the next moment stepping back and thinking about what you've talked about and making it your own. In any case, the families were repeatedly engaged and carried away, just as we were. To this day, reflective conversations have proved to be applicable and useful in many contexts. This applies to clinical work, counselling, teaching, research, planning, mediation, organisations and companies. Since they have taken on so many forms and have so many areas of application, it was natural to stop using the term reflective team and instead talk about reflective processes.

We chose the path called "open dialogue". It was a relief to speak in the open, and it wasn't at all difficult to avoid hurtful speech. Additionally, it didn't take long to realise that speaking politely comes naturally when you talk in the open. What it was that felt so good about this new form was not easy to understand straight away. The understanding of what this new form encompasses has been steadily developed and will no doubt continue to grow and expand. It was the relief of having entered the "open road" that was so liberating. The "open road" is well within the tradition of the road called "practice first, then theory" with the subtitle "practice determines theories".

An example of a reflective conversation

It was the local therapist (LT) who wanted my presence and participation. The elderly couple she was working with accepted it. The LT initially said, "I'm not sure if I should give them advice, or if I should just accompany them in what they are concerned about?" *I thought that my task was to talk to all of them so that LT could find the answer to the question herself. I wasn't going to find the answer.* As the couple listened, LT told me that they (the parents) were worried about their two daughters who were both in their late thirties. One of them, Sara, had been in and out of psychiatric hospitals for several years and had been diagnosed with schizophrenia. She was once a man, but changed her gender in the hope that it would help. It didn't, however, and, in difficult moments, she was preoccupied with taking her own life. Their other daughter, Ruth, had difficulties with food and body weight and had been hospitalised several times when she became so thin that her life was at stake. Her great desire was to be free and independent of others, but her parents were afraid that if they let her go, she would not be able to take care of herself. Neither Sara nor Ruth would listen to what their parents asked them to do. In the conversations LT had with this family, especially when the daughters were present, the atmosphere was often heavy, sad and dejected. *It was easy to see how intensely engaged the parents were. They lived with what they heard.* When LT had said what she wanted me to hear, the couple commented, and LT now sat and listened. She, the mother of the couple said that it was as LT had said, and explained how upset she had been by all the advice her friends gave. They seemed to know better than she did what to do with her daughters.

> They even promise me everything will be so rosy if I just do what they tell me to do. I've become so tired of them that I can't talk to them anymore. I've lost all these friends I've had all these years.

Han, the father, says he's never had many friends, but the man he drives to work with every day also offers advice. "He says, do something for yourself. You need to go out and dance and have fun! I know he means well, and he's kind, but I can't listen to it anymore". He tries to laugh, but it doesn't make the rest of us happy. She says she's not really that worried, because God, the big boss, will take over and help her daughters when she and her husband fall out. He is worried and afraid that they will both commit suicide when they drop out. He sits for a long pause and looks down after he has said this. I've seen this video film sequence several times since. On the film, I can see that he is thinking about the words he himself just said and which he thus heard. He looks deeply affected. Instead of asking if he wanted to convey what he was now thinking, I ask someone about his daughters and the suicide risk. My question took the conversation away from where he was right then to a completely different place. He responds politely to my questions but is no longer "with it". The questions suddenly made him sober up. I ask the couple if they would like to hear what LT and I have been thinking: "She and I can talk together, then you can listen". They're happy to do so, and LT starts by saying that she was very moved by the last thing she heard: "Yes, I suppose it's a matter of life and death". I say that it seemed like there were many people who wanted to give advice. Perhaps the advice itself wasn't the most important thing, but rather the perspective from which the advice came. When her friends gave her advice, they gave it from their perspective and not hers, and when the man in the car gave him advice, the man gave it from his perspective and not his (her father's). Could it also be that it was difficult for Sara and Ruth to get advice from other people's perspectives, and it might have been easier if it came from their own? She and he listened intently to our chat, and she commented afterwards: "From their perspective (Sara and Ruth's) … I hadn't thought about it before … well, they also get advice they don't like…" He said that his daughters wouldn't listen to them, no matter what or how it was said. I didn't ask LT if she had received an answer to her opening question as I took it for granted that she had. The mum had a new idea; he seemed to retain his view of his daughters. Had I followed him more when he talked about his fears for the future, he might have opened up to a different way of looking at his daughters?

To this day, reflective conversations have proven to be applicable and useful in many contexts: in clinical work, in counselling, in teaching, in research, in planning, in mediation, in organisations and companies. Since they have taken on so many forms and have so many areas of application, it was natural to stop using the term reflective teams and instead talk about reflective processes.

Guidelines in the reflective processes

There are often questions about *how* the reflective processes should be carried out. To that, I answer that I prefer to avoid instructing others on how to do it. The best thing is for them to develop their own form, one that seems natural to them. However, I do say that I am happy to share the few guidelines I have myself.

Firstly, I never take it for granted that it *will* be a reflective conversation. Even if there's a group ready to give their reflections, I always ask them first, once the people I've spoken to have told me what they want me to hear: "There have been some people who have listened to us, and who have probably made up their minds about what we've talked about. Would you be interested in hearing what they've thought, or has our conversation been enough?"

Some may be satisfied with the conversation that has taken place, but the vast majority want to listen. In cases where they do want to hear, I point out four possible ways to behave while the group reflects:

> Now do what feels natural to you: (1) you are of course welcome to listen to what the group wants to say, but (2) you may notice your mind going elsewhere. If that happens, just let it happen! You don't have to listen to the group. Or maybe (3) You simply want to rest or (4) Do something else.

I never say what that something else might be, but it opens the possibility of interrupting, leaving the room, etc.

If everything takes place in the same room and the reflective group is also in the room while they are reflecting, I often say to them, not least if some of them are not so used to reflective dialogue: I'm not going to instruct you or myself, but I've gathered some experience over time. When you're talking, I think it would be better for the people listening to you (e.g., your family) if you kept the conversation between yourselves. In practice, this means that you don't talk to the family and don't look at them either. Because if you talk to them or look at them while you're talking, they're forced to listen to you, and they can't *take* their minds off it if they want to. And not until I say so, I say: "But if you can't avoid it, you'd better do what comes naturally. It's about instructing as little as possible".

If I were to take part in a reflective conversation myself, I basically have four guidelines for myself:

1 I will always refer to what I'm reflecting on in the conversation. This is best done by repeating what has been said, and then I will try to repeat, in words and expressions, what had been said. By repeating what has been said, everyone can be taken back to the moment they were in when it was said. For me, it's

important to do it this way to ensure that the conversation being reflected on becomes the context of the reflection.

2 Now I'm only reflecting on what I hear and not on what I see. It's far from certain that the person in question wants what I might see to be seen. What I usually take as my starting point is something that I *can see* is of importance to them.
3 I try to give back what happened to me when I heard what I heard. Usually, it's thoughts, but it can also be an emotional reaction that I can describe.
4 When I convey a thought that has occurred to me, I will reflect in a questioning form: "What if?", "If something should be done, what could it be?", "Who could do it?", "When would possibly the time be right?"

The advantage of questions is that they allow for multiple answers. That's why they're often easy to listen to. I try, as much as I can, to avoid opinions, perceptions and advice, because they can easily be heard as something the listener should think about or do. If what is said differs from what the listener has thought or done, they may easily think that what they have done has not been good enough. That can be difficult to listen to. I make relatively strict demands on myself and avoid characterisations and judgements. That can easily make people think that "they'*re* like that".

If someone in the team comes up with a negative description, a strong opinion or advice, and I'm part of the team, I might be able to ask them: "I wonder what it was like for them (the listeners) to hear that?" or "What was it that you heard that made you think that?" The latter provides an opportunity to discuss whether what was heard could have a different meaning if it were put into a different perspective.

When the team has finished their reflective comments, I will always ask those who have listened: "Would you like to say something about what you've heard, or would you prefer to keep your thoughts to yourself and possibly talk about them later in another context?" It's not at all rare for someone to say that they'd like to think about what they heard, but perhaps most people want to say something. Then the conversation continues from there.

If someone in the reflective group said something that I could sense or see the audience didn't like, I can ask them: "Was there anything that was said that was difficult for you to hear?" If they say no, I won't go any further.

The importance of Greek Kitchen in the Arctic

Through reflective processes, we now had certain practical approaches to how we should relate to people. The open reflective processes felt both democratic and helpful where change was desirable. But did we have a corresponding grasp of how thought could comprehend and understand these processes? What happens when a practice becomes good, and what happens when it becomes bad?

This question was the starting point for the June seminar "A Greek Kitchen in the Arctic" in Sulitjelma in 1988. The name of the seminar signified a desire to realise a particular form of meeting. Almost 25 years earlier, I had been holidaying with my small family on a deserted beach on a small island in the Aegean Sea. Coincidentally, two other couples were holidaying on the same deserted beach in the same week. Unbelievably, both couples were Norwegian, and, unbelievably, we all had many connections between us through family and friends. During my stay, I offered some medical services to some Greeks, as there was no doctor on the island. In return, they treated us to dinner, and we were picked up late one afternoon. The women and children rode donkeys, and we three men walked the 45 minutes it took to get to the village, with its whitewashed houses climbing up the mountainside. We entered a large kitchen, and in one corner there was an open fire where two women were partly cooking, partly serving the food, partly dancing and partly singing. We were seated with the host families around a table in the centre of the kitchen, and the food was delicious: fried small squid, rice and lamb in rolled up vine leaves (*dolmades*) and retsina wine. The smell was wonderful. The heat from the fire was marvellous. The dancing and singing were delightful. And then, suddenly, I realised that the walls were full of people from the village, eagerly watching us and sharing our well-being from a distance. They sat for a while, then got up and disappeared, and new people came, after which these new people were replaced by others. I remember being giddy with excitement and well-being, and thinking: "I would love one day to create a Greek kitchen in the Arctic".

The main question of the seminar was: "How can clinical work with systems, e.g., families, be described and understood?" The invitation to the seminar stated:

> The basis of the seminar is that we want to make it possible to discuss how the work we do can be described and understood. We have invited a good number of people to a dialogue, and we believe that these people will most likely provide different descriptions and understandings of our work. The people we have invited are of particular interest to us because they have been working with so-called second-order cybernetics for a long time, some in theory, some in clinical practice. We hope to be able to describe and explain our work and the work of the other invited clinicians in the light of views from second-order cybernetics. A related question will be whether such discussion can in turn shed light on, and even extend, the epistemology that second-order cybernetics represents.

Based on our own work, we had extensively discussed questions like these: "What is a meaningful dialogue? What is language? What is an alternative meaning? What is change?" The invitees consisted of two groups: epistemologists and clinicians. The epistemologists were Stein Bråten (Norway), Lynn Hoffman (USA), Humberto Maturana (Chile), Fred Steier (USA), Heinz von Foerster (USA) and Ernst von Glasersfeld (USA). The clinicians were the Galveston group (Harlene Anderson and Harold Goolishian), the Milan group (Luigi Boscolo and Gianfranco Cecchin) and the Tromsø group (Anna Margrete Flåm and Tom Andersen).

Three short notes written by the Galveston and Tromsø groups, which were sent out in advance to the participants, included the following:

> We would like to talk together from as many perspectives as possible. We believe that client and therapist develop and create the therapeutic reality together. Since a change (in the client) arises on the basis of a change (through the therapeutic conversations), how can one describe what happens that leads to an improvement or deterioration? How can you describe and explain how you describe and explain? How can the principles of second-order cybernetics be applied in clinical work? And not least: How can the principles of second-order cybernetics be seen in the practical work presented at the seminar?

Prior to the seminar, the ideas of Maturana, von Foerster and von Glasersfeld were discussed in a Norwegian journal. Participants travelling from Tromsø and Oslo had the opportunity to watch the three groups' videos in advance. In addition, all participants had been sent articles written by the epistemologists, as well as transcripts of the videos that the three groups were to present.

On the first day, epistemological principles were presented by the epistemologists and then discussed. They were to represent the basis of the seminar. During the next three days, the three groups' clinical works (video films) were presented and discussed. What happened in these three days was to be the main feature. The seminar, which brought together 160 participants, was organised around shifting conversations: after the six epistemologists had presented their ideas, the participants discussed this in the 32 groups they were divided into, and at the end of the day eight of the groups discussed with the epistemologists. Over the next three days, the clinical groups, one group each day, presented videos of their work, after which the epistemologists discussed with them. The participants in the 32 groups then discussed, and at the end of each day, there was a discussion between clinicians, epistemologists and 8 new group participants each time.

Here are some of the questions and comments from the participants. To the epistemologists: "Can you imagine emotions without language?", "If one cannot predict and does not believe in instructive interaction, what is the difference between a friend and a therapist?", "Does a curative process have to be a two-person process? Are we back to individual therapy?", "The implications of not being a mechanical repairer can be difficult if you belong to medical psychiatry. What does the panel think we should do if our definition of our work clashes with the clients'?"

> Radical constructivism can lead to a weak platform for formulating an ethical basis, values and norms. Some of what is said resembles a radical situation ethics, similar to Jean-Paul Sartre's, in which a relativistic view of knowledge is proposed. That worries me.

To Heinz von Foerster: "Tell us why it's important to value the unpredictable, when it sometimes increases people's suffering?"

> To Harlene Anderson and Harry Goolishian: Do you find the concepts Maturana introduces about emotions such as love, indifference, pain and suffering useful? If so, is it because you think of them as biologically based, or because you perceive them as good metaphors? If you think of them as good metaphors, how are these metaphors different from other metaphors about emotions?

To the Tromsø group: "There are many aspects to the concept of dialogue: understanding, identifying, listening, expressing ideas, etc. What is a dialogue, and what is the difference between a dialogue and 'walking alongside', as you say?" "You say you don't want to intrude on people, and you do so by being reticent. But isn't that kind of passivity a form of intrusion?" "You do what you can to get people to speak for themselves and ask hardly any questions. How is it that you have chosen that way of working?"

What came out of it all? Several reports/articles were written after the seminar. What was unquestionable was that the vast majority, in fact, I think everyone, was enthusiastic. But about what? It was obviously difficult for the epistemologists to recognise the second-order principles in the clinical work. The participants were able to do so to a greater extent. The one who came closest was Odd Arne Tjersland, who started from the idea that "instructive interaction" is not possible. He realised that the Italians were the most instructive and achieved the least. The Americans were not instructive through their friendly and personally engaged puzzle together with the client, where the words were the pieces of the puzzle. The Norwegians weren't instructive either, but in their cautious, respectful manner, they became *too* preoccupied with the formative (the constant discussion with the family about how the conversation should proceed) and thus became a little distant. Ethan and San Martino were more general in their descriptions and not in second-order cybernetic terminology. They felt that the Galveston and Tromsø groups were more open and inclusive of clients, while Milan was more closed and less inclusive. The Italians were, on the one hand, playful, but on the other hand, concerned with how *it was*. The Norwegians were serious on the one hand and mystifying on the other. Harlene Anderson and Harry Goolishian noted in their report that several of the epistemologists were enthusiastic about the fact that the Italians were active, *doing something*, and had the expertise to see what was going on. They also noted that the epistemologists thought the Galveston and Tromsø groups were *too* polite, *too* friendly, *too* accepting and *too* non-instructive. In the final discussion in Sulitjelma, Harlene Anderson and Harry Goolishian made it clear:

> Cybernetic epistemology cannot avoid the underlying metaphors of power and control and thus the inherent linguistic limitations of control theory. This view was countered by Maturana and Steier. Both insisted that cybernetics was a science of human understanding. For us, the fundamental weakness in biological

> epistemology is the underlying theme and metaphor of cellular nutrition and survival. For example, in Maturana's concept of love, hate is not the opposite of love, but the absence of the substance without which we could not survive (nutritional failure). We understand that the basic assumptions of the physical and mathematical epistemologies are expressed by the metaphors of measurement and impact. We recognise that such metaphors not only limit our ability to understand our therapeutic realities but also constrain them. We propose that we abandon the linguistic limitations inherited from biology, cybernetics and physics and begin to explore the metaphors of semantics and hermeneutics.

An epistemology is supported by a particular language, and the fact that the principles of second-order cybernetics were not visible in the practice presented in Sulitjelma was perhaps because the language of second-order cybernetics is neither usable nor desirable for understanding the practice shown. Now, in retrospect, many years later, I can think so. But what was it that made this seminar still remembered so strongly and so positively? I think two elements contributed to that. Firstly, the seminar was organised in such a way that the participants felt that, perhaps for the first time in a seminar of this kind, attention was focused on the therapist. This is a central principle of second-order cybernetics, namely, that we are active creators of the image of those we relate to. One noticed, perhaps for the first time, that attention was thus turned away from the patient, client and family. Secondly, the seminar was organised in such a way that many different conversations and perspectives were included. Few were excluded. Some felt that the atmosphere was "too friendly". A dialogical environment like the one created in Sulitjelma must almost inevitably lead to conversations continuing, both those you have with yourself and those you have with others. I think that's what happened: the conversations continued afterwards.

This was particularly the case for one man, Harry Goolishian. He said his thoughts swirled non-stop and restlessly for the next three months. In October 1988, Harlene and Harry organised the first Galveston conference where the discussions from Sulitjelma continued. Despite the invitations being informal and sent out shortly before the conference, 120 people turned up. This overwhelming interest was probably due to the fact that it was time to reformulate our assumptions about what a human being is and what therapy can be. Harry gave the introductory talk, which he called "A Starting Point for Conversation" and began it like this:

> In the invitation we sent out for this meeting, the words poststructural and postmodern were used to characterise how many of us have begun to change both our ways of working and our theories. Why are these changes in ways of thinking happening so fast, and why is it happening now? Why is it that theories of constructionism are now flourishing, and in so many branches of art and science? Why is it that we've grown tired of what we've been thinking and doing until now? Why is it that the theories and things we have based our work on are fading? As I struggled with these questions, I thought about Ludwig Wittgenstein and his thoughts on language. It would be impossible to understand depth psychotherapy without a

> vocabulary and ideas about the unconscious. It would be impossible to think about love, co-operation, power or romance if we didn't talk about it in the way we do. Without a vocabulary of love, it would be impossible to engage in a romantic relationship. Without a language of power, we wouldn't be able to oppress each other. Without a language of hate, we wouldn't be able to hurt each other.

He went on to say that it is our vocabulary and our ideas about humanity that become so crucial to how we relate to ourselves and others. This language and the corresponding ideas it creates change over time. He then mentioned the different periods: the early Greek period, the early Christian period, the Dark Ages, the Enlightenment, Romanticism, Modernism and Postmodernism. Each period has its own language and ideas. The early Greeks thought that humans had a psyche inside them, which was the real self. The early Christians called this the soul. In the Enlightenment, man was possessed of intellect, reason and logic. In Romanticism, man was capable of strong attachments and had an irrational nature. There are variations in language and ideas in these periods, but there is a common thread: "an Aristotelian thinking" that understands nature and life based on the concepts of structure and its underlying components. Other concepts are form and substance. This leads back to the opposite, namely, Heraclitus's ideas about movement, transience and change, which were rejected by the later Greek thinkers: Plato, Socrates and Aristotle. His emphasis on process, movement and change does not require a separation of subject and object, and there is no emphasis on measurement. His vocabulary and use of it promote a view that the world is always on the move. It is a view and a representation that does not require a separation of us from nature; it does not require grand explanations or final conclusions. For Heraclitus, the world was an ever-changing balance of conflicting tendencies. There was no private or subjective world. It is this second Greek "path" that postmodern, poststructural ideas bring us back to.

In December 1988, Harlene Anderson and Harry Goolishian wrote the article "Human Systems as Linguistic Systems: Preliminary and Evolving Ideas about the Implications for Clinical Theory" in the journal *Family Process*. The article begins by saying that through their practice, which had taken place over many years with many different types of problems, often very large ones, they had been constantly reminded of where they fell short: that their (and their contemporaries') theories and practical activities had not been enough. This has been the driving force behind their search for new theories and new practices. In other words, many years of pondering over stubborn and unresolved clinical challenges lie behind what they eventually came up with and discuss in the article. They mention five premises. They can certainly be described as five ontological premises:

1 Human systems are language-creating and, at the same time, meaning-creating systems. Conversations determine the social organisation (the system), and not the other way around; conversations are a result of the organisation (the system).
2 Meaning and understanding are created when people interact with each other and exchange their thoughts and experiences about the same event or phenomenon.

3 A therapeutic system is designed and defined by the "problem", rather than by a social structure that defines and reshapes the problem.
4 Therapy is a linguistic activity that takes place in what we call therapeutic dialogue.
5 The therapist's task is to create space to enable a dialogical discussion. In this context, the therapist is a participating observer and leader of the discussion. The therapist's task is to take part in this process in such a way that the problem, through the dialogue, is dissolved, and that the therapeutic system is thereby dissolved.

Systems can be understood in two completely different ways. This can create a dilemma for thought. One is linked to a dominant idea in the social sciences, whereby a system can be described and understood in terms of its structure and roles. The other way is to understand the system based on ongoing interactions; the organisation and structure are a result of these local and timed interactions. In the first approach, the system is described not only in terms of structure and roles, but also in terms of stability, hierarchy, power and control. This general social theory, on which the authors believe most psychotherapies are based, is well described. Order and stability are maintained through control from above. To maintain the stability of the system, the relationship between the parts of the system and the processes taking place must be such that the structure and the parts remain unchanged. You could call this an "onion theory". Each system lies on top of another like the layers of an onion. One layer is subordinate to the layer above, and all serve the order and stability of the whole. The individual is surrounded by the family, the family by a larger system, this larger system by society, and so on. The imposed restriction of role and structure becomes an armour that exists independently of people and contributes to the order that society calls culture and civilisation. Problematic behaviour, pathology and deviations are seen as inadequacies in roles or structure. This is caused by something wrong in one of the layers, and it is transferred to the layer below. Something wrong in the family structure that is reflected in the family's individuals may be one example. Therapy should try to repair this social defect. Concepts such as empiricism and objective reality are linked to the "onion theory".

The second way of looking at things, which the article began with in five points, contrasts with the "onion theory". Human life and human meanings are created through what happens between people: togetherness, conversation, collaboration, coexistence, etc. Language is central to everything that is done together, and the author says that such language consists of more than spoken words. They believe it encompasses all the forms of exchange that can take place between people.

Kenneth Gergen points out that meanings are created in interaction, for example, in conversations, with others. This social meaning-making process has been called social constructionism. The language exchanged through conversations includes active expressions, and language is not just a linguistic activity but also a social one. Language is what makes it possible to describe reality, and that description makes it possible for us to relate to reality. This view is in line with Bateson, and in contrast to the idea that we have direct access to and contact with reality. Although second-order cybernetics is far from being comparable to the "onion theory", both use some of the same concepts, namely structure and control.

The article by Harlene Anderson and Harry Goolishian was finalised six months before the Sulitjelma seminar. It turned out to be a very important article that has attracted a large readership over the years. I remember that Harry Goolishian took a "stand" against cybernetic language, including metaphors, structures, interventions and other technical and mechanical concepts. This was also a rejection of a sociology that embraces a model in which social organisation is based on social roles and social structures that build on each other in layers, and which defines a problem as a structural defect. People are not determined by the structure of their own, their family's or their local community's organisation, but by the conversations they take part in and the language they use to express themselves.

In 1990, the June seminar in Melbu was therefore about "language systems". Once again, we tried to link practice to theoretical perspectives, this time the language perspective. Kenneth Gergen and Jan Smedslund from the University of Oslo were invited, and the Houston-Galveston group (Harlene Anderson and Harry Goolishian) and the Tromsø group (Pål Talberg and I) showed video-recorded conversations. As was the case in Sulitjelma in 1988, it was again difficult, when studying the conversations, to retrieve the elements that were claimed to be essential based on the theories. But the "paradigm shift" that we had been experiencing for several years began to become more comprehensible.

Harlene Anderson and Harry Goolishian organised a conference in 1991 in Houston called "Psychotherapies for the Next Millennium", which clarified matters further. Kenneth Gergen attended, and John Shotter[1] became a new acquaintance. He emphasised that human being was not a collection of internal structures or an inner core within the person. He invited us to consider that the conversations taking place between people and the language they use make them the people they become. This was a big leap in thought, and not least a heavy challenge for those who held high and visible positions in academia. That's why there was a major new conference in Lofoten in 1993, which essentially centred on the new language perspective. It was a broad and wide-ranging elucidation of, and great support for, this "new", as far as I was concerned. I was still to take part in a psychiatric/psychological world, both practically and academically. This world was neither aware of nor interested in these new perspectives, preferring and applauding "the old" instead.

I've thought a lot about these "rational" conferences we organised. It turned out to be difficult to fully integrate the practical work into them. Some of the most important aspects of the practical work were not included in the "rational". For example, the handshakes we exchanged (a handshake *and* the look that followed the handshake) with people, how we used our eyes when we tried to see and how we listened when the other person tried to tell us what they wanted us to hear. In 1993, I was one of many people asked to contribute to a book under the auspices of a social constructionist organisation. We were free to decide what we wanted to write and how. It could be a story, a game, a language image or whatever. What follows is my contribution. Is the contribution a sign that the rational superstructures had become too big and heavy?

A simplified guideline for the conversation aimed at analysing and finding a solution to a mental health problem. Useful for both individuals and multi-person systems (families)

The key to solving the presenting problem is first to identify what the person themselves, and possibly their loved ones, have done to solve the problem. It is the attempted solution that is the real problem. This first requires clarification of what the presenting problem is. This is a surprisingly difficult task. It is also important to clarify who has the problem. It is surprising how often this is not clarified.

Please be kind

The perception of reality held by the person(s) seeking help should be the starting point for your work. Avoid interpreting their views and opinions about what their reality (and problems) are and avoid moralising.

Notice things you like about people. If there is something you dislike, say to yourself: “If only I knew that person better, I would understand what makes it necessary to act that way”. Get used to thinking about the positive ripple effects a particular way of behaving can have, even if it is labelled as problematic.

It is important to be aware of a help seeker’s often intense resistance to effective help. This resistance can emerge at any point during the analysis of the problem and its conditions. The goal of the resistance is to make the helper ineffective, and the helper must know how to act in order not to be outmanoeuvred by this resistance. Go with, rather than against, the resistance. Never try to fight it, you will only increase it. Accept it, and even signal that you are willing to accept *more* resistance. In doing so, you reduce the resistance.

Who finds the situation problematic?

This is the first and perhaps most important clarification. The importance lies in clarifying whom you can expect to collaborate with. Problem-solving requires a change in the way people behave towards each other. Since such a change is both demanding and uncomfortable, it is unlikely that anyone other than the person(s) experiencing the situation as problematic will be involved in a (treatment) partnership. You may therefore not include the identified patient (IP) in the collaboration if he perceives himself as problem-free. In other words, make sure you know which of the people sitting opposite you thinks the situation is problematic.

Clarifying questions in this context can be, when several people are present: “Which of you finds this (= the problem presented) problematic?” When one person is present: “What was it that made you come here?”

If the answer is that others suggested it, it should be clarified what the person's position was on this proposal. Is he/she here because he/she has been persuaded? Is he/she here because he/she thinks he/she should be? Clarify whether the person is here now because they want to solve the problem. If this is not confirmed, there is no reason to continue working with this person unless he/she perceives another relationship as problematic for him/her. In that case, however, the starting point will be different from the problem presented.

What is problematic?

If several people are present, for example, an entire family, ask this question first to the person who seems to be the most influential. Of course, it's difficult to ask this question so early in your meeting with the family, therefore, trust your intuition here. Then continue asking in the order you believe reflects each individual's level of influence. The question could be: "Tell me what you, from your point of view, find problematic". Let the respondent answer as freely as possible. Note the way and the words they use to describe the problem. Later, it is useful to refer to their problem using the same words.

Bring out all the problems for the individual

Avoid redefining the problems. Take the person at their word. When all the problems have been presented, ask the person(s) sitting opposite you to focus on one problem. It is common to ask them to focus on the most important (or biggest) problem.

The next step is to characterise the problem. In what way does it occur? When does it occur? Does it occur in specific situations? Which other people are present? It may be appropriate to spend a certain period, for example, two weeks, recording the problem; time, place, situation, countermeasures, etc.

Get to the start of it all. What kind of episode did it all begin with? Try to find out what else happened to the person and their loved ones (i.e., the person's family). Did something occur that led to changes in the composition or function of the family? Were new family members added or dropped, or did relocation, accident, illness, etc. occur? What aspects of the family's relationships were put to the test by this event? What speaks in favour of, and what speaks against, solving the problem? What will the consequences be if the problem remains unresolved? Bring out all your thoughts and fantasies about how this could affect the individual's and everyone's social functioning.

What would the consequences be if the problem was solved? For example, it could lead to other new functions that *could* be burdensome and responsible; it could also be that something is lost and, for example, lead to loneliness. Use your imagination when describing this! You may find the question useful: "Amidst all these difficulties, are there still some bright sides that you would lose if the problem were solved?"

Perhaps the most important thing is to get to grips with the values or norms on which a person/family bases their actions. Problem-solving requires a change in the ways of acting in the problem situation. Since this way of acting can only take place within the values and norms with which the person/family has framed their life, it is important to find out where this framework lies. Problem-solving (= change) will often require this framework to be expanded.

This framework is a synthesis of the values on which the individual and the family as a whole build their community. Such value frameworks can be exemplified by the following: the family must stay together and never break up; certain topics are taboo and must be kept quiet; certain ways of acting must be suppressed and controlled.

This part of the conversation provides an opportunity to redefine the content and meaning of the problem. In other words, the problem can be viewed from several new angles. This can be utilised in further work to change the way the person in question relates to the problem. In this way, you can imagine that the change in problem-maintaining behaviour is already underway.

When weighing up the pros and cons, you will get an impression of how important it is for the person to solve the problem presented. It is hardly appropriate to get heavily involved in an issue where the person's eagerness to solve the problem is lukewarm. The more critical a situation is, the more the person will want to change it, and the more you should become involved.

What are the solutions tried (so far)?

After the person(s) has (have) defined the problem he (they) perceives as the biggest (and possibly also defined a positive goal), your next task is to find out what he and his loved ones have done so far to solve the problem. This part of the task is divided into two:

Firstly, you need to get a description of what has been done as a solution attempt, and secondly, you need to understand the person's reasons for solving the problems in the way he has tried so far. Regarding the first, namely, what has been attempted, it is particularly important to highlight how the person has behaved towards other people. This behaviour does not come out of nowhere but is underpinned by what the person tells himself he should do and influenced by how others, especially those closest to him, behave towards him in the problem situation. What the person tells himself that he should do is linked to the idea of what might happen if he does not do what he does.

Based on the information and observations you have made so far, you step back to find ways to break the ongoing attempts to solve the problem. The ongoing attempt to solve the problem is also a way of relating to each other. It is this way of relating to each other, your communication, that must change if the problem is to be solved. Communication can be understood by observing how they relate to each other when you are in their presence.

Make up your mind about how they approach each other. Who do you think has the most influence? Who seems to initiate or change the topic of conversation? To what extent do they agree or disagree with each other's positions? How do they behave when they express disagreement? Are there alliances between any of the parties? If so, between whom?

It's the communication they have that prevents them from getting out of the presenting problem. It may be enough to break the communication at *one* point with one of the people. This is best done with the person who believes they have the most control over the ongoing communication.

Note

1 John Shotter came to mean a great deal to Tom Andersen's later development from the early 2000s until his death in 2007. This collaboration was not textualised in the same way as other collaborations Andersen had. Four references have been added to the back of the book, in which John Shotter describes and discusses Andersen's work in light of his philosophical musings. There is also a reference to a conversation Anne Hedvig Vedeler had with John Shotter in 2007 about her collaboration with Tom Andersen, shortly after his death.

Part 3

The place and importance of language

Chapter 6

The power of words – yes, the power of expressions

In the autumn of 1989, something happened in the practical work that I discovered and understood in my mind three years later. The conversation in which it happened was filmed, and I have watched it many times since. This means revisiting the therapy described earlier, where a local therapist and an elderly Jewish couple were present. They had two daughters who both lived difficult lives. One of them, who often thought about taking her own life, had also been diagnosed with schizophrenia and, to have a better life, had an operation to change from a man to a woman, unsuccessfully. The other had been diagnosed with anorexia, and her condition had threatened her life several times. The therapist was unsure what to do, whether to give advice or just follow the family wherever they wanted the conversations to go. The elderly couple listened with intense participation. There was one phrase that had come up in their conversations recently, and that was "Tsores". "What does that mean?" was my question. "It's a Yiddish word", said the therapist, and the daughters' mother in the background said: "It means problem". "The word is bigger than that", said the therapist, "it means both grief and pain". There was a silence in the room, and the therapist said: "I've suddenly gone blank", I said, "You were just talking about the uncertain fate of your two daughters, and then you said the word Tsores. Can you find your way back to your thoughts, or are they going to be gone?" "They will be gone", she replied. "So Tsores is a meaningful word?" I asked, and she nodded yes. "The sorrow that is in the word, is it a silent sorrow?" "Yes", she said. "Is it a lonely grief, or the grief you share with others?" "It is that which is shared with others". As she said these last words, the strength of her voice diminished, almost to the point of breaking, and a very seriousness entered the conversation. The feeling that arose in me at that moment was a bit like the one you feel in your body when you step on the first thin layer of ice on a puddle in autumn and the ice breaks. "And the pain in the word?" "It's that helpless feeling. They want something to happen to their daughters so that they can take care of themselves after their parents have passed away". "Is the pain a pain in the heart or a pain in the head?" "It's a pain in the heart". Between each question and answer, there were long, silent pauses and the parents sat and listened in intense tension, as if the words hypnotised them. Me: "What is the nature of the pain?" (…). Therapist: "I don't know, but it's that helpless feeling you have when you so intensely

DOI: 10.4324/9781003357742-11

want to do something but don't know what it should be" (…). Me: "Is it like reaching for something, but not getting there?" (…). "Yes, it's a matter of life and death", said the therapist (…). All four of us were gripped by the sheer power of the words, and we all sat for a long time thinking. For my part, I felt that the words had gained power over me and embraced me, and I felt that, in this almost sacred moment, I had to tread carefully with the questions. The words were no longer inside me, but I was inside the words. "Yes", said the therapist, "the parents probably think all the time about what will happen after they pass away". The mum said she wasn't too worried because God, "The Big Boss", would take over, while the dad was afraid, they'd both commit suicide. These questions, which "examine" some of the words that are expressed, came to light and thus could not be grasped by thought until a couple of years later. It was now obvious that the listener should *see as much* as she or he listens, perhaps seeing even more than listening. On several occasions, I have said that you should listen as much with your eyes as with your ears.

The transcript that follows comes from a meeting after I had become aware of these new questions. The local therapist requested my presence in the meeting, and the client, Wanda, accepted this request. Early in the session, she told me how upset she became during the past week when her mother called and asked her to visit her mother's mother, Wanda's grandmother, who had been hospitalised two weeks earlier. "How on earth could she wait a whole week before visiting her own mother?" Still upset, she explained that she herself had been ill two years ago. She had a sore throat with a high fever and had to stay in bed. The fever and the pain in her throat disappeared, but she continued to stay in bed for six months and finally realised that it was more than a throat infection. She realised that she felt sad. Me: "How did your family look at you … did they think you deserved to ask for something for yourself?" Wanda:

> (…) I don't really know (…) I don't know if they look at it that way (…) I think that (…) well (…) look at (…) I think that the family I grew up in (…) we were expected to be able to rely on ourselves (…) to some extent rely on ourselves (…) independence was the big word in our family (…).

Me: "Rely on yourselves?" Wanda nods yes:

> Yes, independence was really the big word in my family (…). *Both times she says, "independence was the big word in our family", a sad look comes over her face, and as she says this, the pitch of her voice drops, and I think it might be of interest to investigate that word further.* (…) and I feel that it was something that I incorporated into my life (…) I have (…) no (…) once they weren't responsible for me anymore, it (…) it was no longer an issue (…) I mean they don't talk about it anymore (…).

Me: "But it's still there?" (…)

Wanda: … it's like (…) to ask about (…) when I was ill my sister finally came to me and said she wanted to call my mum (…) you have to get her here, she said, and my mum came and I thought it was difficult, because then my dad was left on his own (…) it was very (…) it was awful (…) you see I got the feeling that (…) I was causing (…) I was causing (…) I was in my own crisis, and then I was causing a crisis for others (…). It became a kind of chain reaction (…) something bad happened here and led to something bad somewhere else (…) it was pretty awful (…) everyone was a bit affected by it, I don't know what others would have done (…) I mean, in an ideal situation (…) I don't know (…) by the way, I don't know what would have happened in an ideal situation (…) if (…) I don't know (…) if, if (…). *All the time she speaks intensely and is strongly engaged in what she says and hears* (…) Me: "How was the word independent expressed? Was it in the open or was it implicit?"

Wanda: "Well (…) straight out (…) literally".

Me: "Literally? The word independent?"

Wanda: "Yes".

Me: "Was it how you were going to be independent, or was it independence in general?"

Wanda: "We were going to be independent (…) they wanted us to be independent (…) and" (…).

Me: "So, as time went on and you got to know the word and let that word become part of yourself, what do you see if you look into the word independent?"

Wanda: I don't like it, personally I don't like that word very much (…) partly (…)". *She says this with an attempt to smile while shaking her head slightly from side to side* (…).

Me: "Do you see anything that (…) say more (…) what do you see that you don't like?"

Wanda:

> Well (…) talking about loneliness is so hard for me (…). *She starts to cry and brings her hands up to her face while her shoulders sag a little forward and down* (…) You see (…) this was something I tried not to think about so much (…) uhm, yes, I think the word independent means to be alone (…) and for me to be lonely (…) to be alone (…). *She is crying as she speaks* (…) it's (…) uhm (…) what that word (…) we talked about being independent and finally I said: Don't use that word about me anymore (…) it reinforces something in me that I don't like (…) having to do everything myself (…) having to (…) I've always felt it's been pushed on me (…) for me (…). *She stops crying* (…) What I would like to do (…) I don't think there is any strength in being independent (…) I don't think there is any strength at all (…) I mean to manage on my own (…) I actually don't think (…) I don't think (…) I mean (…) manage myself (…) I don't treat others like that (…) but I do treat myself like that (…) but in the end I said: I'm not independent (…) I'm not independent like you think (…) I may have grown up with that idea (…) but I don't believe it now (…). *She straightens up and strikes out with her hands and her voice is stronger and she speaks faster* (…) I think you should be supportive (…) I think you should do things together (…).

Sometimes you must look for expressions other than words. I've previously described the conversations with the five women, where the grandmother, Elisabeth, preferred to sit and listen from the start. The eldest daughter, Maren, wanted to talk, as did the local therapist. Elisabeth's youngest daughter, Trine, said early in the conversation, "I'm just a driver", which gave me the impression that she might prefer not to talk. I wasn't sure what Maren's daughter, Elisabeth the younger, at 13, wanted; to listen or to talk. There was a lot of laughter in the room. Maren, Trine and Elisabeth the younger laughed out loud, especially when Elisabeth the older said something. When the phrase "a black cloud" came up, I asked the therapist if everyone was ready to talk about what was in the cloud, while the four women listened and had their own inner reflective conversations about what they heard. The therapist, who said she tended to protect Elisabeth the younger, believed they were ready and said that Elisabeth's father, Maren's first husband, had abused Maren so horribly and so much that Maren ran away from him when Elisabeth was a baby. They were both still angry with him, Elisabeth because he never allowed her to meet Maren, and because he never helped her take care of Elisabeth, either with money or attention. But Maren was also scared. She was afraid that if he met Elisabeth, as Elisabeth herself wanted, he might take Elisabeth away from her. As they talked about their anger towards him, Maren said that they were also angry at and fought with each other; she, Elisabeth the younger, the two other children she had later, and Elisabeth the elder, who lived near them. However, they didn't fight with the person they were angry with, but with someone else. For example, there was a lot of tension between Maren and Elisabeth the younger, but Elisabeth the younger didn't take it out on her mother, but on her grandmother.

At this point, about 25 minutes into the conversation, Elisabeth the elder, who had remained silent until now, began to move and wanted to say something. In a loud voice, she spoke directly to her granddaughter and said, among other things, that she didn't like her anymore and recounted a couple of episodes that were unfavourable to Elisabeth the younger. There was a lot of laughter in the discussion of difficulties and anger, and the laughter came from Maren, Trine and Elisabeth the younger, especially every time Elisabeth the younger said something. The laughter eventually became so loud that it was difficult for me to hear what was being said, and I knew that this could make me irritated if it continued. For the time being, it helped that I said to myself: "If their laughter is the only way they can be present, how would they cope in this situation if I stopped them and took away their laughter?" That question to myself helped with patience. However, it was so disturbing and so hard to hear that I chose to talk to the therapist for a second time while the four women listened and had their own inner conversations about what they heard. "I noticed that there was a lot of laughter in the room, even though what we were talking about was quite serious. I've always wondered if this laughter could speak, what would the words be?" While the therapist was looking for an answer, I asked, "Are they happy words or sad words?" Without hesitation, the therapist said that they were sad words, which led me to ask, "Is it so sad that we should avoid talking about it?" The therapist became uncertain and said for the second time that she had a tendency to protect Elisabeth the younger I remembered what she had said early in the meeting: "They were stuck, and they didn't know how to move forward", and asked, "If it's not possible to talk about this sadness, how are you going to move on?" "Yes, that's it!" she exclaimed. "That's where we're stuck!" Elisabeth the younger started to move around on the chair again in preparation to say something, but I stuck to the conversation with the therapist and asked several times if it was wise to talk about the sadness. In the end, Elisabeth said, "We are here to talk, we can no longer keep it under the carpet just to protect Elisabeth the younger. If we don't get it out in the open, it won't go well for us!" There was both anxiety and laughter as she spoke, and immediately afterwards she told us that she had cancer and that the outlook was bleak. It was obviously something everyone knew but couldn't talk about for various reasons. It would have been easier to fight. Now that it was finally said, we could talk about it. Trine couldn't bear the thought of losing her. Elisabeth the younger said she couldn't afford to lose her grandmother because "she's been here for me all these fourteen years!" Elisabeth the younger found it hard to imagine that she, who had stood on her own two feet since she was 14, would now be dependent on others. "And mum is scared too", said Maren, "as we all are". The therapist noted that they had tried twice before to talk to each other, but that it hadn't worked. "It had something to do with me", said Elisabeth. "I was so angry at my fate. But now that I can admit that I need help, I can participate". Trine said she now understood what Elisabeth the younger had been through and what her crying, acting out and difficulty concentrating were related to. "I didn't understand it before either", said Elisabeth the elder. "Even mum hasn't understood it", said Elisabeth the younger, after which her grandmother said, "Mum is always the last to know".

On another occasion, I was meeting the board of an organisation in another country. They found it difficult to grasp my way of thinking and working, so they asked if I could show them instead of telling them. When I asked if anyone had anything they wanted to discuss, Lena jumped at the chance. She said she wanted help with something she was dealing with at home, namely working with a family the child welfare authorities had ordered them to work with. She worked at a child and adolescent psychiatric outpatient clinic, where she was manager, supervisor and therapist. In this case, she had all three functions at the same time. The family consisted of a mum, a dad and four children. A ten-year-old boy had his mother from a previous marriage and the other children, aged seven, five and three, had their mother and father together. During the two years they had been working with the family, the parents had separated, and the father was allowed to visit his three children from time to time. The allegations against the family were that there were violence and abuse between the parents and from the father towards the four children. Suspicions of incest were also hinted at. The team, which worked exclusively with the mother and not the father, had asked for the court's help in issuing a judgement whereby the mother or therapists could ask the police to intervene and arrest the father when he was dangerous. The court had rejected this twice, much to the team's annoyance and despair. Things had become particularly bad in the last two weeks. Firstly, two weeks ago, when the father had been on a road trip with his three children, as he drove back to the children's home and saw his ex-wife walking on the pavement with her ten-year-old son, he accelerated the car and drove it onto the pavement to run them both over. His own three children watched from inside the car and saw that he was fortunately unsuccessful in his attempt. Lena spoke clearly and easily and with great intensity. I remember imagining a man who might one day succeed in murder, and it sent a chill down my spine. What was even worse was that a week ago, the little ten-year-old boy had run out into the street where there was heavy traffic to be run over and killed. He had tried twice without success. To protect him from his stepfather and himself, the adults had sent him far away.

Lena's negative description of the husband made me realise that I couldn't take it for granted that she would be able to talk about him. I therefore concentrated the conversation on how there could be protection for the children, the wife and the team, which consisted of four women. Only after thirty minutes did I try to talk about him, and fortunately, Lena could bear to talk about him. They had never met him, and I thought that THEN they must really be afraid of him. However, being a man myself, I knew that dangerous men become even more dangerous if they are excluded, so I began to discuss with myself in an inner conversation whether there was any possibility of including him. But I kept the idea to myself, of course, as I thought she might not like it. I therefore asked: "This man who shows so much anger and brutality, does he only have angry and hateful feelings, or does he also have other feelings? Does he have mixed feelings?" "Yes", Lena said, "but at the moment he turns them all into angry feelings". I was relieved that we could talk about him and his feelings, even if they were of the negative kind. I returned to the safety aspect before picking up the conversation about the man again: "I understand that boundaries have to be set, or a fence has to be made around him. Does it have to be done exclusively by others, or can he be part of it himself?" The ideal would be if he could be part of it, Lena thought, but now that was probably unthinkable.

> Then you also said that he has mixed feelings, but that he currently converts them into one feeling, namely anger. And it goes without saying that he makes others afraid. Which of the other emotions would have made people less afraid? For example, if he knew more sadness or fear, would people be less afraid?

"Well", said Lena, "if he showed more sadness than anger (…) that might help the situation". She sat there thinking. I realised that I was starting to get a little anxious myself, and to curb my eagerness, I asked a question for my own sake: "Do you have a feeling that your colleagues working with him have any faith in him, or have they given up on him?" Lena answered, "I think they've given up on him". Me: "Okay, so they've given up on him. But, if there was someone who hadn't given up on him and was able to talk to the sad part of him, that might be something?" (…). Lena stayed in her own thoughts for a long time. Me: What kind of man is this? How would you talk to him so that his sad side comes out? Another long silence (…). Lena: I don't know, I don't know (…) I don't know if he feels that anyone is listening to him (…), or if he has ever been heard? Me: "(…) and if there was an answer to that, maybe nobody would bother to talk to him? Is it possible that this man spends a lot of time alone and therefore feels lonely?" Lena: "There seems to be a lot I don't know about him. After all, we haven't met him". Me: "No, how on earth would you know everything? So, it's hard to know if he's available?" Lena: "I don't know, but I don't think he's available". Me:

> The reason I'm asking these questions about this man who threw his car onto the pavement to run over his ex-wife and ex-stepson while his own children watched, was it pure hatred that drove him to this, or could there also be other emotions in it? I wondered about that. If there was some sadness in the terrible event (…), could you reach that sadness by talking about the act? I simply wondered about that.

Lena: "At the moment he denies everything". Me: "Or a similar incident, an incident he can talk about (…) if that incident could be discussed so that his dilemmas came up, maybe you could ask him: Who can you go to and discuss your dilemmas with?"

We left off there, and I wished her all the best in her future endeavours. The next week, I learnt from someone else that when Lena had returned to the team, she had spoken in his defence. She suggested that she and another new employee should try to meet him. They did, and he was happy to meet them, and he was punctual for the calls. However, one day a secretary came and said he was behaving in a way that scared her. They told him this and asked him to stop acting like that. He did so. While the conversations with the man were going on, the ten-year-old boy handed in a tape to the police in which he had read that not only had his ex-stepfather abused him, but also his mother. The court intervened and issued a judgement that placed all the children in foster care. Two years later, Lena reported that the children were flourishing, the father was making great progress and there was talk of giving him custody again. The mother was perceived as not yet ready to regain parental rights. Five years after the above conversation, Lena saw in a newspaper that the husband had been named "Father of the Year" in the small town where they now lived. Lena made the connection between that and the conversation we had had five years earlier.

A separated couple were unhappy and angry with each other. She was bitter and angry; he was bitter and sad. She wanted him back, but as a changed and better man. He didn't want to come back, but he couldn't go through with the divorce either. Their seven-year-old son, Erik, was angry when he was with his mum and sad when he was with his father, where he was also unhappy. I said to him, "I noticed that you used the word sadness about your son and sadness about yourself. Are there more emotions in his sadness than just sadness?" Him:

> I think there are mixed emotions. I think he's also angry sometimes, and sometimes he's also scared. During the two to three days, he's with me, he starts by being sad, but after a few hours it goes towards anger, and I can see it already on the first day.

Me: "If his anger could speak, what would the words be?"

> Oh, many things. Why did you leave me? You don't act like I'm the most important person to you! And it's hard for me because my father left our family when I was seven years old. What worries him a lot is when he realises that I'm seeing another woman. He's afraid that I'll have another child and that he'll be completely left out. That's why he always wants to know where I am.

She and I then had a long chat about her desire for him to change. "(…) but he is like that, and his problem is that he can't change". After this meeting, I later learnt that he thought enough was enough and wanted to go through with the formal divorce. A few weeks later, she realised that she had to give up both him and her desire for everything to change. The following year, she had started studying at a university and had also begun to flourish.

A couple in their early forties were unsure whether they dared to get married. They had periodic explosions, and there was a distance between them. It happened when she thought he was getting so close that she felt "eaten up", and he was getting close because he was afraid of being abandoned. She thought that she either had to give herself up and get close to him or give him up to fulfil her wishes for independence and an interesting and rich profession. He wanted to get close to her but was afraid that closeness created the explosions that drove them apart. "It's when we don't really know how close we should be to each other that war breaks out. A war of fear. But we don't talk about the fear". Me: "Is the fear in the mind, or is the mind in the fear?" He gasped in astonishment and sat for a long time looking at the wall and repeating to himself, "Is the fear in the mind?" (…) Me: "Or the mind in the fear?" (…). Another long pause, during which he thought intensely and she looked at him in intense tension. "Fear is in the mind (…) well, maybe a little bit both ways". Me: "Is that fear just fear or are there other emotions in it?" Him: "I don't like to be occupied with either anger or fear. I shut down". Me: "If you shut down, maybe you haven't been able to see into the fear. If it were ever possible to investigate fear, what do you think you would see?" Him: "Then I might see myself abandoned and frightened and weak, and see something that would make someone even more lost". Me: "So you wanted to see that you were abandoned and weak, and that someone left you?" Him: "Yes, I wanted to see everything that wasn't attractive about me". Me: "Does that mean you have to be attractive not to be abandoned?" She leaned towards him and gripped his forearm warmly: "If that happened, you couldn't be more attractive!"

He walked around for two months with the question, "Is the fear in the mind or is the mind in the fear?" swirling in his head. There were no more explosions after this meeting, and they got married a year later.

A woman was concerned about peace and was asked the question: "Is peace a big or small word for you?" "It's big", she said. "If you were to walk into the word peace, what would you see and hear?" "Then I walk into a meadow on a late summer afternoon. The sun is coming in from the right and there's no wind, and I hear music". "What music?" "Mahler's Second Symphony". "What part of it?" "The final movement, where the choir comes in". "Are you with someone, listening to the music?" "No, I'm alone…" and she started to cry. "If you could have someone to be with you, who would it be?" She knew the answer. "If you brought a picnic basket with food and wine, what kind of music would you choose to bring?" She knew the answer.

A therapist wanted me to interview him in front of the workshop participants so they could see, and not just be told, how the work was done. I knew he had experienced something unpleasant the day before and asked if this was the right place and time to talk. He thought so, and he told me that the day before he had received a call from the prison where one of his clients had been incarcerated. Her mother, who was dying and in great distress, had asked her daughter to end her mother's life. She did so and called the police, who took her to prison. When he told this story, he spoke in all seriousness. "I was in the same situation myself two years ago", he said, "my father asked me to do the same thing, and I couldn't do it". He wept quietly as he spoke, and the audience sat in silence. Everything he said included the words "I can't bear to see anyone suffer", and when he heard his own word "suffer", he burst into convulsive tears, and I thought, "We shouldn't touch that word, it brings too much pain!" That's why I pulled out other words he had just expressed: "…I don't want to be a burden to others". Me: "Which others is it important not to be a burden to?" We had a long chat about it. The pain receded, and the crying stopped. It seemed that, in this moment, it was better to talk about others and not about oneself, and for the time being, to keep the word at a distance.

Peter, the local therapist, wanted me to meet a couple in difficulty, and he wanted me to be active and himself to be passive. However, it turned out differently. He talked to them for half an hour, completely immersed in their situation. The couple, in their early fifties, had approached Peter a year earlier because their daughter had made a dramatic change. From being every parent's dream, beautiful, intelligent, sociable, good at school, friendly and helpful at home, warm and happy when they went on holiday together, a year ago she had completely changed. She was now 17 years old and no longer wanted to live at home. She had moved into a commune where there was free sex and drugs. She dressed like a punk and had stopped going to school. She had sent a present for her father's birthday but not for her mother's. This had hurt her mother immensely. He said, among other things, that he was a man of "understatement". She said that perhaps she should have challenged her daughter differently, and "(…) perhaps I myself should have been challenged in my perhaps rigid way of being a mother".

When Peter suddenly, after half an hour, realised that I was present and invited me into the conversation, I asked, "What do you want me to do here?" It came fast and hard from her: "I want you to challenge me!" I must admit that I was not a little flabbergasted and said to myself within a couple of tenths of a second that now YOU were challenged. Let's see if you can stand up for what you believe in! Don't try to figure out WHY she said this. Just listen to what she says! Me: "How do you want me to challenge you? Friendly or tough?" Her: "Not friendly". Me: "With understatement or without?" She: "It's up to you!" Me: "Then I choose without understatement". She: "Yes, by definition it has to be if it's going to be tough!" Me: "What's tough?" She: "I won't know until you've done it!" Me: "What would the opposite of tough be?" The man whispers, "Tender", and she laughs a little and puts both hands on the back of her neck as she says, "Yes, tenderness". As she puts her hands on the back of her neck, I think that this is either sad or painful to talk about.

When someone places both hands on the back of the neck, the collarbone is lifted and fixed so that the chest muscles can more easily raise the chest. And the need to be able to lift the chest may be related to the fact that the movements in the stomach stop when the stomach muscles are tensed. When the movements in the stomach stop, what feels sad or painful can feel a little less sad or painful. With these thoughts, a great seriousness comes into the conversation, and it influenced me to say to myself: "For God's sake, don't interrupt her when she's talking!" Me: "Have you encountered tenderness?" She: "Yes". Me: "So you know what it is?" She: "Yes", and drops her hands from her neck. Me: "Tell me more about that tenderness so I know what to choose as the opposite". She raises one hand and slowly rotates her open hand as she says, "That would be to open windows and doors gently to let fresh air in". Me: "So it's tenderness, so when I'm going to do the opposite, I shouldn't open windows and doors gently?" She: "If you're going to do the opposite, the roof should fall in, and the walls should fall out and windows and doors should be blown out! If you're going to build something new, the old must be demolished first!" Me: "Are the foundations going to be removed too?" She: "Foundations are just illusions, they're myths!" Me: "Is the new house going to have no foundation?" She: "This can be built on other illusions!" Me: "What could it be?" She was thinking intensely, and it came precisely, with a long time between: "(…) telephones (…) CDs (…) cars (…) cups of tea (…) glasses of red wine (…) grass (…)". Here she became a little less intense, so I asked, "What kind of grass?" She: "Long, brown, dry grass and short, green, juicy grass". Me: "For walking in or sitting down in?" She: "To roll around in!" She continued with other illusions, and they became more and more vivid, for example, a teddy bear.

I asked her husband, "What are your thoughts?" He said, "I didn't understand anything!" No, I thought to myself, I didn't either, but that's not so important, because she herself understood enough. When she had "built" the new foundation, I asked her how the new house would look from the outside, and she told me about the shape and the windows and doors and colours. She told me about the flowers and trees in the garden. Then she told me what kind of rooms there were inside: two study rooms, rooms for guests, the bedrooms, rooms where the guests would eat. It became detailed. I was the one who finally had to ask if there would also be a room for the daughter, and she said, "Yes, a room for her too". When the house was built, she grabbed her bag and asked if I was interested in seeing some holiday photos. There were a lot of them, from when her daughter was seven up to when she was fifteen. All three of them were in the pictures, smiling, wearing clothes with fresh and bright colours on holiday in her home country. Each picture had a long and happy story that felt wistful in the current situation. Two weeks later, she wrote a letter to Peter saying that the conversation was of the utmost importance, namely, to be able to go from layer to layer without having to follow a plan, just letting what came, come.

Two men, both with life-threatening AIDS, were deeply engaged in a conversation with Peggy Penn and me. They were married and had come to Peggy and her then-colleague, Marilyn Frankfurt, a year earlier for help in getting a divorce. One, Joe, a dance teacher, thought the relationship limited him, and the other, Richard, an architect, accepted Joe's wish. However, as one tangle after another was resolved, the desire for divorce disappeared. On this day, Peggy wanted me to talk to them so that she could follow it all from a distance. Early in the meeting, they told me about their interests in music, especially singing. They also told me that they had worked a lot with the words "to be alone". For Joe, the meaning of the word was that he could go behind a door, close it and be left alone. For Richard, the meaning was to run behind a door and close it to keep an attacker away. Richard also said relatively early in the meeting that Peggy had mentioned at the end of the previous week's meeting that there was a word that had been suppressed, namely, death. All four of them had probably thought a lot about it but hadn't talked about it openly yet. When they now opened about the word, it turned out that both had had many thoughts about suicide, either doing it separately or doing it together.

"But we can't do that", said Joe. "In a way, we become a role model for those who come after us". Joe was very ill and clearly tired, and we could sense a strong desire to die. We could almost hear his inner voice saying, "Let me go!", just as we could almost hear Richard's inner voice saying, "Please don't go yet!" These were the two voices we were supposed to listen to and talk to, without taking sides. The more tired Joe seemed, the more Richard cheered him up: "Of course you can't do everything you used to be able to do, but there's still a lot that can bring you joy!" "Yes, but I've lost so much", Joe replied. "It's like my identity has been ripped out of me. My thoughts are whirling round and round; they won't stand still". "That illustrates my point", said Richard. "A lot of good can come out of mental activity, which you have so much of!" Joe's shoulders slumped a little, and he said, as a police car outside whistled past, "What I want is to go out into a desert and let all the voices quiet down and disappear. That's the kind of being alone I now look forward to". There was a deep sigh as he looked intently at Richard. My eyes now followed Richard, who seemed to be in pain, and I said to him, "Is it hard to hear that Joe wants to go?" Richard said, "Terrible! Intellectually, I can take it, but not emotionally". There was a great silence in the room. "When the thoughts that he might be gone come to mind, reading a poem or listening to music helps. But it doesn't stop the tears from falling". Then he straightened up and sped up his voice and said, "I know that these are just thoughts. Ten years ago it would have been serious. But not now. It helps me to read about the miracle stories of chemotherapy". I nodded in agreement *and thought now it's important for him to find the pace and his words that dull the pain.* "The fact that he talks like this is because he has seen so many of our friends pass away". I nod in agreement. "Besides, this way of talking is an expression of anxiety and depression". I nodded in agreement. "And it is again an expression of illness". I nodded in agreement. "He's just started taking the happy pill, and it will soon take effect". I nodded in agreement, and Joe said it had started to work. "When I look at the situation that way, I can get past it and move on". I nodded in agreement, and said, "Maybe strong bonds last forever?" "Strong bonds (…) last (…) do you mean our bonds?" "Yes, maybe they never go away?" "I solved that a long time ago!" he then said with great intensity. What Joe and I need to talk about now is what to do with our ashes. I'd like something to go to each of our families so they can bury it somewhere where they can go and say, "Here's Uncle Joe' and 'Here's Uncle Richard". Both he and Joe moved their hands as if shaking a cocktail mixer, and both laughed, and Richard said, "I'd like the mixed ashes to go under an azalea bush". Joe leaned his head forward and shook it slowly from side to side. "What would that be like for you, Joe?" I asked. "It's sentimental", he said. "Not for Richard", I said, and Richard nodded his agreement. Joe's face filled, in a hundredth of a second, with sadness, and he said:

> No I understand (…) I can go along with it (…) it's just that if there are any remnants of spirituality in the ashes, I don't want it put on a mantelpiece. Besides, when I realise how little Richard vacuums, the ashes will probably stay here for a while.

We all laugh, and we all know that right now it's better to laugh than to cry. Then Joe said to Richard, "What if I die and you get a new lover?" "If you go first, I'll take care of your ashes until I come back". Thinking about the music we talked about earlier in the lesson, I asked Richard, "If that asalia were to blossom (…)". Richard interrupted, "It will be the biggest and most beautiful asalia in the whole cemetery (…) the lushest (…)", and I continued, "When it blooms and there's singing and music in it, what will the lyrics be?" "No, no", he said, "it won't be a song. It will be chamber music. Vivaldi's Four Seasons (…) no, it's going to be Beethoven's Pastoral Symphony (…) the morning sequence (…)!" Peggy asked Joe, "What music do you have in mind?" He looked at her with the big eyes of a clown; cheerful and sad eyes. "It must be a disco flashback from the seventies!" Everyone laughed again, and Joe said, laughing, And at my funeral there will be a big party (…)". Peggy said, "Lots of dancing!" (…) Joe continued, "(…) Yes, lots of dancing. And those who still know how to fuck will get a little extra company for it!" We all laughed. Richard talked at length about how much he and all their friends would miss him when Joe died. Then Joe asked me, with his big eyes filled with laughter and (…) grief, "What are you thinking, Tom, just before we finish?" "Well, I don't know if I can find the words, but there will probably be beautiful words and sad words", I answered. Richard whispered softly, "Thank you (…) it must be hard for you to be struck by such a tragic story as we have!" "No, I don't feel beaten, I feel moved", I replied. Richard: "Well, beaten is an American jargon!" "Well", I said, "beaten is a short word. Moved is a longer word. This meeting will probably be with me for a long time. Most likely for the rest of my life". "Thank you", Richard whispered, while Joe's big eyes express the same. As we walked out onto Lexington Avenue in the November rain, we had the feeling that during the meeting we had gone from life into death and through death into life again. We met six months later. Joe read a love letter to his mum. Richard read a letter to humanity in which he hoped that in the future there would be room for many different types of marriages and families. I took the opportunity to ask what the most important thing is we, who call ourselves therapists, should do. Joe answers quickly, without hesitation, "You will listen to and witness our stories".

Chapter 7

The meanings of expressions in treatment and research

This chapter deals largely with self-evident truths, many of which you will undoubtedly agree with, but which you nevertheless fail to consider in your daily life. It is conceivable, as Ludwig Wittgenstein says in the quotation above, that what is discussed here is so right in front of our eyes that we do not notice it. The chapter is an attempt to put the obvious together in a hopefully useful way. Although it consists of obvious things, it turned out to be very demanding to write. Perhaps this is because the ambitions were set quite high. I have tried to create it in such a way that it can serve as an overview for those who are trying to understand both the differences between different practice activities and the differences between different research activities. One of the difficulties with the chapter is that it contains several elements that are, in a way, intertwined. To understand one element, you must first understand the others. Therefore, the elements mentioned first will easily be left hanging in the air, since understanding them is dependent on understanding the others, which come later. The chapter may therefore have to be read twice, and perhaps only when you read it the second time will it make sense. It has been difficult to avoid many repetitions.

The elements in question are: (1) Preconceptions, which I call basic beliefs, (2) Language and the social significance of language, (3) The importance of the language community in relation to both practice and research, (4) The pre-linguistic, that is, the importance of bodily functions for intellectual functions, (5) The process that leads to the creation of meaning, and (6) Key aspects of the "human", such as "what is a human being and what is the world they live in?". The importance of language in the development of the individual is central here. The chapter represents thoughts that have been collected and organised over time – thoughts that have perhaps first and foremost come from practical work, but also from discussions with professionals and lay people, and, of course, from reading. I would say that the main framework for these thoughts is the practical experiences, as they are "known on the body". The chapter can therefore perhaps be regarded as "known through the body" musings. The experiences came first, then the reflections.

The practical experiences referred to here are primarily from various working relationships, where the emphasis has been placed on the relationships being of benefit to all those who are part of them. At the very least, they must not harm or

DOI: 10.4324/9781003357742-12

offend those involved. Damage is not something that can be easily seen and formulated. Rather, it is something that only the person who is injured feels through their body, and which they themselves may find difficult to point out and articulate. Injury occurs, for example, when no one wants to hear what you are saying, or when those present are not interested in trying to understand what you are saying, or when those present do not believe what you are saying. This chapter is therefore largely formulated from experiences of certain types of relationships, namely, the open conversations where everyone could hear everything that was said if they wanted to, or not listen if they preferred. Everyone could talk if they wanted to or keep quiet if they preferred. Everyone could talk about what they wanted to and was exempt from talking about what they didn't want to talk about. Everyone who talked could find their own way of talking and use the time they needed to say what they wanted to be heard. The others had to be present to hear and witness what was said and, if necessary, then say what they heard did to them.

Certain relationships were avoided, namely those where one party stands at a distance to explain the other's situation, and where one party tells the other how they should or should not live their life. If the relationships I am reflecting on had been different from those I took part in, the experiences would, of course, have been different, and the content of this chapter would have been somewhat different.

Text, speech and words

By means of the text in this book, I am handing over to the readers something that has been, and still is, important to me as a writer. The words and the text convey descriptions of two realities: one is the practice of treatment that you have now read about; the other is the exploration of the meaning of this practice, which you will soon embark on. All descriptions are simplifications of what is being described, including this one. The two realities were far richer than the text can recreate for the readers or for myself. Words give meaning by making you relive something you have experienced before. The words in the text therefore create meaning that becomes personal to each individual reader. You understand the text in relation to what you've already understood. I must therefore be prepared for the text to recreate the two realities in different ways for different readers. Paradoxically, the text can also contain more than what is described. Within the framework of Paul Ricoeur's philosophy of language, it can be said that language can also have a surplus of meaning in relation to the event it is supposed to formulate. Linguistic ambiguity can be found in both words and sentences. It can be intentional, as in metaphors and symbolic language, but is often unintentional in everyday language. The event contains more than the meaning, and the formulated meaning more than the event. The result is a dialectical relationship between event and meaning that calls for interpretation. To bring the reader as close as possible to the two realities in which I took part, I have endeavoured to use everyday, ordinary language – the language that ordinary people share. In other words, I have endeavoured to avoid any expert language. When one and the same person writes a particular word, reads the same word silently, or reads it aloud to someone else, the word can quickly take on three different meanings for that one and the same person. Also, if I, as the author, were to read the book aloud to the reader, the author, as the reader, would most likely realise that a word or two would touch and move them. For the time being, I will call this the mystery of the spoken word, which arises only in a conversation where another person, or persons, are present, watching and listening to the reader or speaker. In this chapter, language, words, expressions, and conversations will be discussed in more detail. What has been written above is simply to clarify that every text is a simplification of what you are trying to describe.

Fundamental beliefs

Within the so-called hermeneutic tradition, it is common to refer to a basic assumption or a basic belief as pre-understanding, after Martin Heidegger, or prejudice, after Hans-Georg Gadamer. The idea is that one is *not* neutral when forming an opinion about something. We inevitably carry with us certain general ideas about what is "characteristic" of what we are facing. For example, if the task is to understand another human being, our basic ideas about what a human being is will determine how we understand the individual before us. For the past three to four hundred years, it has been common to believe that what a person says and does is "fuelled" by an "inner core" that exists within them. With such a basic belief, you will take what a person says and does as the external, representative signs of that person's inner core. If you also believe that this inner core constitutes an essential part of the person's uniqueness, you can, based on what this person says and does, interpret what and who he or she is. Ultimately, all of this is based on the fundamental belief that there is an "inner core". This raises a question: how would you be able to understand this same person if you held a completely different fundamental belief? This is one of the big questions.

The hermeneutic circle

This little sketch indicates that one's basic beliefs influence how one understands, for example, another person. Regardless of one's basic beliefs, when encountering another human being, one may experience something one has never experienced before (Figure 7.1). This new experience of what is "human" will be fed back into and may nuance or even change your basic beliefs. This process is called the hermeneutic circle. Already here, one can add a basic belief about the basic belief: one can be uncertain or convinced of it. Thus, the sketch is slightly expanded.

This invites you to take a stand, which I am happy to do. I *think* it's good to be uncertain about your fundamental beliefs – not least because you are then prepared to maintain your vision and possibly revise your beliefs. If you're *convinced*, it's easy to put on blinders and see *only* what you've already seen.

It is important to note that it is *not possible not to* have a fundamental belief. The challenge for all of us should be to find out what it is when we make up our minds about this or that.

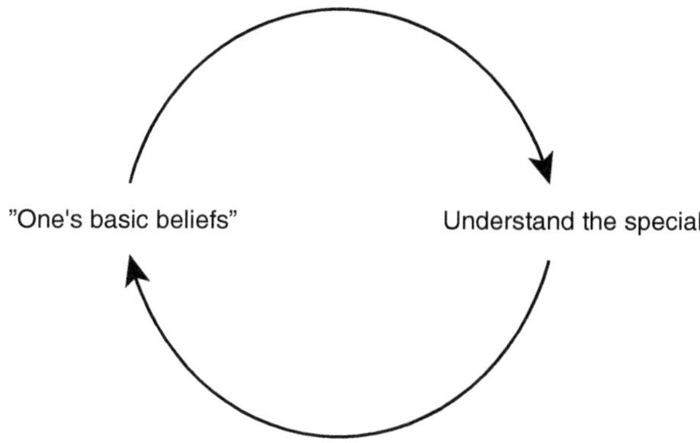

Figure 7.1

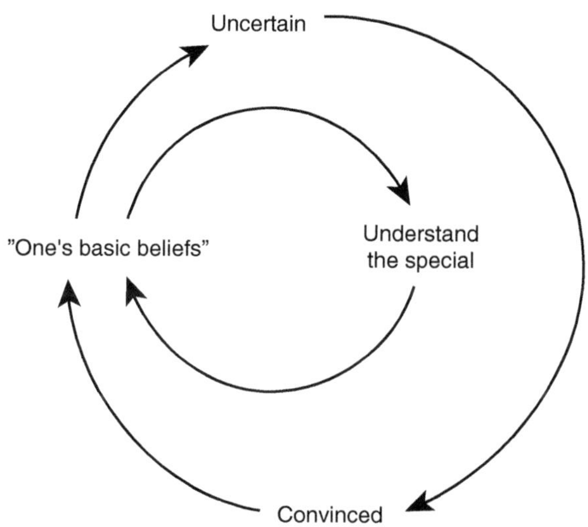

Figure 7.2

A balance – how do you strike a balance between believing *enough* to be able to take part in daily life, and doubting *enough to* be able to change or even give up your belief when the time comes? In this chapter, it probably shines through that the author's faith is quite strong. If it feels that way, try to understand that the faith is *temporarily* strong – not lasting.

Five basic ideas about language

The simple sketch above can also be used when thinking about how language can be understood and what language means. In the following, I will point out some basic ideas about language.

It is a condensed presentation compared to the sources it relates to. The sources are also my own experiences from practical work in the so-called reflective processes and in collaboration with physiotherapists in Northern Norway:

1 Language consists of expressing (showing, giving) signs (symbols). The bodily activities that accompany the use and practice of these signs are part of the expressions. The signs can be sensed, as something you hear, see, are touched by or even smell or taste. Although words, the sounds we call words, are the most common language signs, the others must not be forgotten. All signs are expressed, and the expression is a bodily activity. When the bodily activity takes place in relation to others, the expression becomes part of a social interaction. Language then becomes a social activity.

   There are many forms of expression, and bodily activity is found in all of them:

   - Dance is a physical activity.
   - Speaking (talking), singing, and acting are sound and bodily activities.
   - Painting involves paint, a canvas, a brush, and a bodily activity.
   - Sculpting involves clay or stone, tools, and a bodily activity.
   - Writing and drawing involve a pencil, a paper and a bodily activity.
   - Mechanical writing involves a computer and a bodily activity.
   - Measuring involves an instrument and bodily activity.

     The last two forms of expression are mechanical and limited by technical possibilities.

2 The expression carries meaning. The meaning lies *in* the expression – for example, *in* the word, not under or behind it. The expression is meaningful because the perceiver is reliving something they have already experienced. Among other things, words acquire meaning by being related to and illuminated by other words in one's vocabulary. The product – the painting, the sculpture, the music, the theatre piece, etc. – also carries a meaning, but one that is different from the activity of expressing oneself. If you see a sculptor at work, you see both the sculpture that gives meaning and the activity of the working (expressing) sculptor that gives the sculpture meaning – sometimes violent, sometimes careful, sometimes thoughtful, sometimes spontaneous, etc.
3 The expressions come first: then comes the thought. As Harry Goolishian always said: "It's all about talking so we can find out what we're thinking!" You search through your repertoire of expressions to find the most suitable one. When the expression is found and given, the meaning is formed; for example, the clear thought or the vague idea.
4 Language is both *informative* and *formative*. When a person expresses themselves, they tell something about themselves – both to themselves *and* to others. The expression is therefore informative. However, the expression also has another side, – the formative side. This means that you become who you become

through what you express. Based on my fundamental belief, it is not only opinions that are shaped, but the whole person. You don't do something nice because you are nice; you become nice when you do something nice. The sculptor can be violent one second and gentle the next, thus creating two different sides of themselves.

5 Language "casts a spell". The formative power of language is so great that it moulds the mind and can change one's basic beliefs. If you say enough times that "he or she has a lot of aggression in him or her," you could be bewitched into believing that something like aggression exists; for example, either as a thing or a structure. You could be bewitched into believing that aggression is something you *have*, as something stable over time. And you could also be bewitched into believing that aggression is an internal component of the person. Another way of expressing the same phenomenon could be: "He or she got angry when he or she was exposed to this or that". If you continually express yourself in this way, you may be bewitched into thinking that people get angry because they react to something linked to certain events at certain times.

What is important to realise is *that it's impossible not to* be bewitched by your own language.

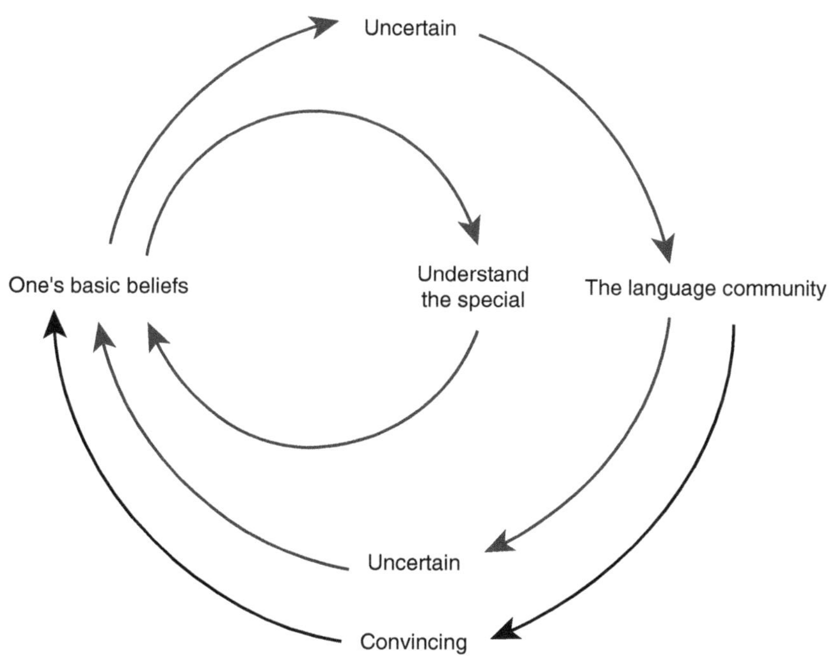

Figure 7.3

To be bewitched by your own language is to be human. The interesting thing is to find out *what* kind of language you are bewitched by, *and in what* way, and then ask yourself whether there is another language to be bewitched by, and how that language might exist.

The understanding of language discussed here is a crucial basis for the arguments in this chapter. The time has come to nuance the sketch that has already been shown:

One's language is regulated and shaped by the everyday language community one is part of. The extent to which a community accepts and includes many forms of language – or does the opposite, namely excludes all but "the right form of language" – is therefore crucial. Based on the above about the bewitching power of language, each person's daily expression will shape their fundamental beliefs. A community that includes many forms of language will allow for many and varied fundamental beliefs. In a community where only one form of language is accepted, basic beliefs will easily become standardised. The language community takes on significance in relation to our uncertainty or conviction. In the sketch, I have suggested that one can become uncertain about the conviction the community sends out, and then one naturally sends one's uncertainty back to the community. The "convinced" community rejects the uncertainty and, of course, only sends back a stronger conviction. The "uncertain" community tends to accept and discuss the uncertainty.

The impression and the meaning of the impression and the expression of the meaning

The impression of one thing or another leaves a mark, like a footprint in the wet sand. It can be something you see, hear, taste, smell or feel, like a brush against your skin, a bump against your body or a grip on your body. The impression is given meaning by comparing it to something you have experienced before. The meaning can be formulated in words, captured by thought, and expressed, for example, like this: "There's a mountain over there", or "There's a man standing on the side of the road".

However, the meaning can also be a vague bodily sensation, and the only thing one can express is, for example, "this is uncomfortable, where "this" has something to do with the mood in the room, but where the mind is unable to grasp what "this" is. Sometimes the meaning can be expressed as "Ugh!!!" or "I got so nauseous…" without being able to articulate what is going on.

It may even be that you can't find a single word, but that you just go and throw up.

When the impression is a word, and you hear a word, the word can be given meaning by reliving something you have experienced before – either a taste, smell, image, sound, brush against the skin, bump against the body or grip on the body. These re-experiences produce different reactions, from bodily pleasure to bodily discomfort, which we call affects, feelings or emotions. The meaning becomes corporeal and can be said to be related to the fact that, for example, the word, that is, the sound, initially touched the person's ear and then, when the word was heard, moved the whole body – indeed, the whole person. The moment thus becomes quite rich in content, namely impressions, bodily movements, and opinions that are expressed. In a way, the moment becomes movement, a moving microcosm.

Naming and labelling

You *give* the child a name. You do not name the child. The child's name is a gift.

But there are many things you *put* a name to, and then the name is not a gift but perhaps rather part of a conquest. A close friend of mine, the theologian Ebbe Reichelt, and I enjoy sitting at my holiday resort, looking out to sea, discussing and speculating. I would like to quote something he wrote about our speculations in a festschrift to me:

"The creative power of the word" is a basic theme in human religions. It was also a recurring theme in our deliberations. A key area related to this is that of naming as a way of making oneself "master" of what one can name. The nameless anxiety is then the opposite. What we name (or diagnose), we can control. In the Middle East, a deposed king could be given a new name by his conqueror and was thus transformed into a relatively faithful vassal. Of course, God could not be given a name. He had to reveal it Himself and allow it to be used only on very special occasions. The misuse of God's name was therefore a grave sin – an attempt to lord it over God. Tom also reacted quite adequately when I tried to name parts of his property. According to human primal instinct, I threatened to make myself king of a rock just outside his cabin by naming it "Table Mountain". If anything, I should have known how insulting that was. Tom's annoyance was a good illustration of today's theme. Words are also a bridge to reality that brings reality into our consciousness. But the strange thing is that the better words convey reality, the more they threaten to replace it. Words become a wall against reality that shuts us out from it. And the better they are, the worse they are. Zen masters constantly shake their disciples by stepping on "sacred" symbols and words that prevent them from experiencing reality. Diagnoses produce something of the same result (Reichelt, 1996, p. 142).

What is it that we make up our minds about and put a name to?

Paradoxically, we have begun to form an opinion about something before we have met it.

The basic belief contributes to that. What we say, do, and believe is simply a continuation of what we have already said, done, and believed. I will try to say something general about the world we live in – about nature, the people around us and ourselves. When I read what Ludwig Wittgenstein wrote, it made me realise that the world is divided into parts that we both see and hear and know *are* there, and that we can therefore know *what they are*. Examples include a mountain or

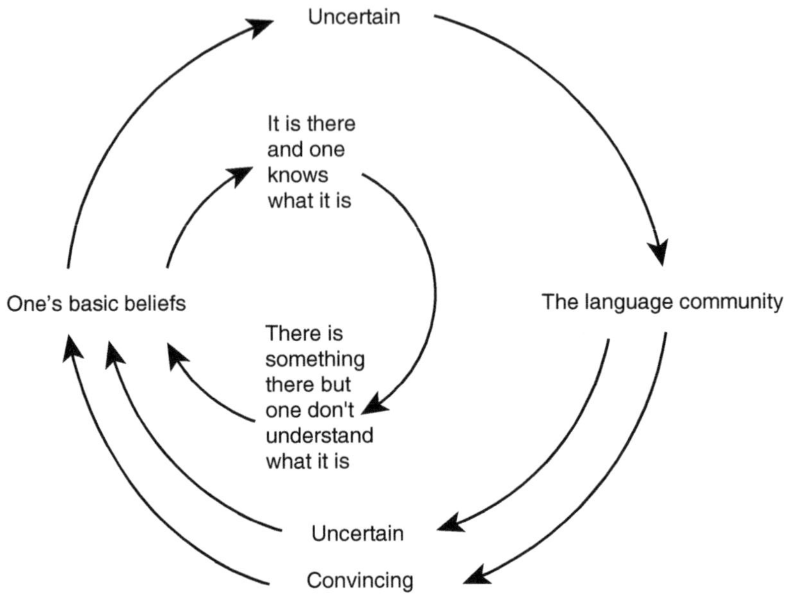

Figure 7.4

the man standing on the side of the road. We can see and touch both the mountain and the man on the roadside. We also know that another part of the world is there, but we don't understand what it is. For example, we can see, or rather sense, that the man standing on the side of the road feels discomfort. Perhaps pain, shame or humiliation? We can sense it, but we don't fully understand what the man's pain or shame, or humiliation is. Partly because we don't have a language to describe it. But we sense that there is "something" there, and we usually find out how to relate to the situation where this "something" takes place. We are affected and moved by what we sense in such a way that we find out how to relate to it. The kind of knowledge we are talking about here, and which I will discuss later, is what I would call relational and bodily. Much of what we are faced with in relation to other people is of this type, both when the relationship is called treatment practice or research practice – namely, that part of the world we "feel in our bodies" and do not understand with our minds because, among other things, our linguistic formulations fall short. Once we have named what we sense, it is easy to believe that what we have named exists. But does it exist? We should answer neither yes nor no. We should say that we don't know. At this point in the chapter, we find ourselves in a strange situation. Since the linguistic formulations fall short, it becomes difficult to talk about, write about, and understand these important aspects of life, both for therapists and researchers.

Our little sketch can now be expanded a little more:

Some of what is there remains unchanged over time. The mountain stands there in the same way – winter and summer, in storm and calm. But the man at the

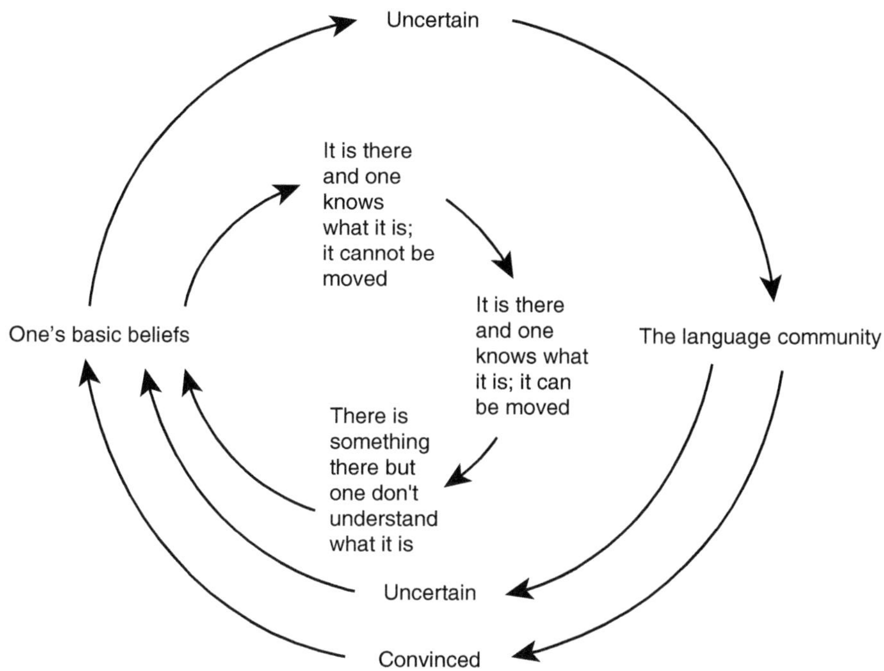

Figure 7.5

roadside changes with time and circumstances. He cannot, for example, stand by the roadside indefinitely. Every now and then, he must go home to lie down and sleep. His expression also changes, for example, from happy to sad, depending on what he is exposed to. The world that has so far been divided into two parts needs to be divided into three, and we need to expand the sketch a little more.

What we know is there, we can touch – both the mountain and the hand of the man at the roadside. The mountain cannot be moved. But the hand can. It can either be clenched or open; it can be at rest, or it can be extended for a handshake. The "something" that is there, but which we do not understand – for example, what the man's handshake expresses, and to which we give the name "warm" or "firm and trusting" or "reserved" – touches us. We cannot touch this "something", the meaning of the handshake, in the same way that we can touch the hand. We can only be touched by it.

You give your hand to the handshake. His hand is in your hand. The handshake is created when the hands meet. But the "warm" handshake – can you feel it in your hand? Or is it seen in the other person's eyes? Or is it felt when the other person's body moves and adjusts to the handshake?

The sketch needs to be nuanced:

From now on, the word touch must be perceived in two ways: both touch and touching, to bring out the two possible meanings of the word – the literal and the emotional (bodily).

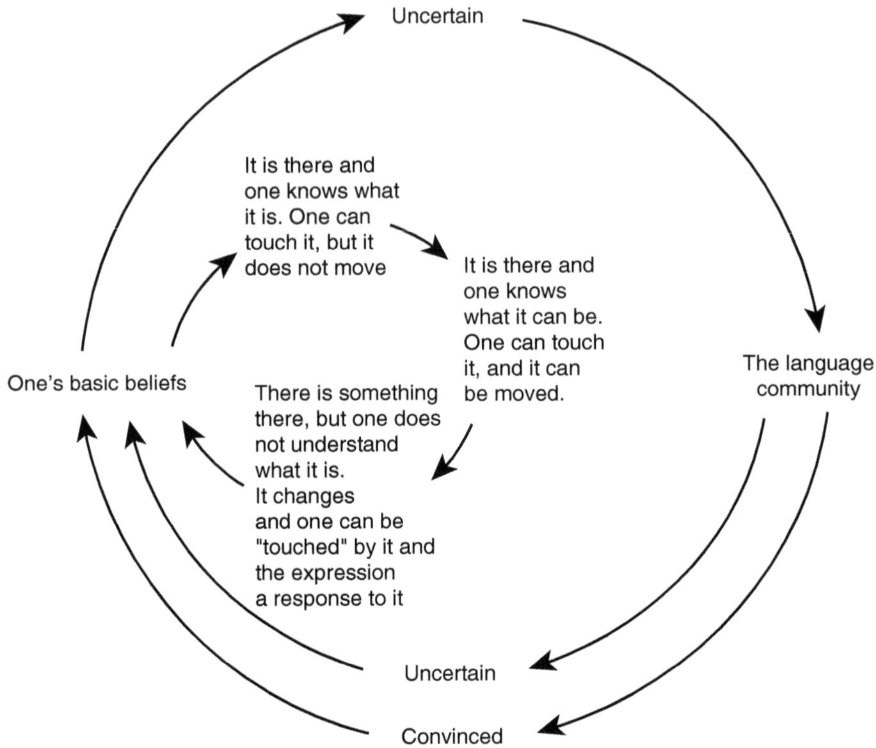

Figure 7.6

It is, or, it could be, or we don't understand what it is

At this point, it is important to remember that a linguistic description of something and this "something" are not the same thing; the description and the described are two completely different phenomena.

J - B - V: I create my Description of the World (Reality).

The description connects us to the world (reality), while at the same time standing between us and the world (reality). It is by means of our descriptions that we relate to the world ("reality"). Some say: "My descriptions *are* my realities". Since our descriptions are shaped by our language, some say that "my language enables, on the one hand, and limits, on the other hand, my 'realities'". The description "his warm handshake", as it is read on paper or heard when someone says it, is not the same as what one senses when meeting the man's hand in a warm handshake. The sketch, as it is now, can illustrate that there are three different statements or three types of linguistic descriptions we can have about the world we live in. One part of the world is that which is there and which we can touch with our eyes or hands or questions or measuring instruments, and then explain. We can even come back and repeat our touches. This represents the part of the world where we can say: this is how it is, for example, that the mountain is so and so big and it is so and so steep. That's what it is.

The other part of the world is also there, and it can also be seen or heard or measured, for example, seizures with rapid heartbeats. The heart can be both calm and restless. Some people have long-lasting reactions after stresses they are exposed to. Others do not. We should therefore say that people can react like this to stress, but not necessarily. We can therefore understand what this might be. In this lies the possibility that this other can be different. It is what it is at the given time and in the given context.

The third part of the world includes something that is there, but we do not understand what it is; we only sense that "something" is there when we are touched by it. We sense the beauty of the mountain when we look at it from afar, and we sense the power of the mountain when we walk in it.

Our sense of this "something" tells us how to relate to it. We feel it in our bodies and know how to deal with it. Feeling the body is simply seeing and hearing and tasting and smelling and feeling touch against the body, either as a stroke or a bump or a grip, and then also feeling your own body's reaction to this.

Explain or understand or sense

Phenomena in the first part of the world can be both explained and predicted. The knowledge gained is certain and can be generalised, that is, it can be transferred to other contexts and to other times. This type of knowledge can be pursued and achieved in the physical sciences. Phenomena in the other part of the world can be understood but are difficult to explain and predict. This knowledge changes with context and time and can therefore be generalised to a limited extent. Moreover, it is assessed based on its applicability rather than its correctness. However, there is a certain relationship between understanding and explaining. For example, misunderstandings may need to be cleared up to understand what the other person means. An example is: one person explains, "No, it wasn't her handshake, it was his handshake I was talking about", and the other says, "Oh yes, yes, then I understand". Phenomena in the third part of the world can only be sensed, that is, "felt through the body", and the paradox is that when you try to grasp this part with your mind, for example, by naming it, you will easily lose contact with it, that is, lose the sense of touch.

What happens when we put a name to what we're facing?

I have now come to perhaps the most important point in the chapter. As Ludwig Wittgenstein put it, our linguistic formulations "capture" and "bewitch" the mind: "Philosophy is a struggle against the bewitchment of our understanding by the means of our language" (p. 109) and "'That's *the way* it is' – I say again and again to myself" (1953, p. 113). Since expressions, including words, have formative power, we can come to describe what is there – and what changes with time and context in such a way that we are "bewitched" into believing that it is unchangeable. For example, expressions such as "he'*s* aggressive" or "he'*s* vulnerable to stress" or "he *has* a firm handshake" can easily lead one to believe that he *is* like that. The idea that a person has "characteristics" is sustained by our linguistic expressions to ourselves, and this language that "belongs" to the linguistic community we are part of thus shapes our beliefs about this.

What's worse, our linguistic descriptions of the "something" that we sense is there, but don't know what it is, can lead us to believe that this "something" exists, as if it were a thing. On a par with a fact. In psychiatry, there are countless examples. In relation to a person who is in a "psychotic crisis", we sense that there is "something" there, but we do not understand what this "something" is. This "something" can quickly be labelled and described as "he's sick". If the crisis lasts long enough, we may begin to say that "he is schizophrenic" or "he has schizophrenia".

Ludwig Wittgenstein reminded us of many things, including to be careful about labelling what is there, but which we do not understand what it is. With his words in mind, I would therefore like to say that it is just as dangerous to say that things like character traits exist as it would be to say that they do not exist. We simply don't know if they exist. It is just as dangerous to say that schizophrenia does not exist as it is to say that it does. We don't know, and that's what we should say.

It can be dangerous to put a name to this "something" that is there, but that we don't know what it is. The name can begin to determine the future. I have previously described the major upheavals in psychiatry in northern Finland:

> Until 25 years ago, psychiatric care in northern Lapland was synonymous with confinement in mental hospitals far to the south. The family members cared for there were often regarded as the living dead, as they remained there forever, cut off from their loved ones. As a result, there is a long history of fear and distrust of psychiatry in the communities and a tradition of caring for the "insane" for as long as possible and solving difficult problems within the family. Families would rather hide their problematic members and keep their secrets than let society hide them in a closed institution.
>
> (Seikkula, 1996, p. 112)

A woman in her mid-teens was restless and ran around a lot. She also had difficulty concentrating her thoughts. A professional "explained" to her that she had probably been abused. The mum, who knew the alleged abuser from another context, accepted the professional's assumptions. Some of the family members adapted their lives to this understanding of reality, and the family disintegrated. In a conversation with the young woman five years later, she said that there came a day when she no longer knew whether the idea of abuse came from the professional or from herself, and there came a day when she no longer knew whether there had been abuse or not. I understand this example to mean that when an idea that was originally a fantasy one had for oneself; an "inner voice", is expressed openly with the help of an "outer voice", what is expressed can have great power. It not only transforms an idea into truth but *can* also create a vivid experience of something that has not happened.

What happens if you say: "A psychotic crisis is normal". It is likely that those affected by the crisis will participate in it with their own normal expressions, even the "psychotic" one. Perhaps one should say, "We don't understand what it is, but we can certainly try to find out how to deal with it". But how are we supposed to find out what it is, if it's possible to find out? Perhaps ask those who have experienced such a crisis and let them tell us in their own language? What happens if someone says: "A psychotic crisis is sick"? Perhaps you would then think that it needs to be treated in a special way? Perhaps by specialists? If that's the case, what words and phrases will you look through to understand, or even explain, it all? Will they be words and expressions that the "psychotic" feels at home with or alien to? If you must "understand" an incomprehensible situation using a foreign language, what will happen? Perhaps it's better to say, "We don't understand what it is, but we can try to figure out how to deal with it". But how can we understand what it means to describe the incomprehensible in an incomprehensible language? Perhaps we should ask those who have experienced such a situation first-hand and let them tell us in the language they prefer.

The problem can arise when our prejudices, or what I call basic beliefs, are not "seen through". *Before* we begin studying and describing one thing or another, our preconceptions have "decided" whether what we are facing can be explained or understood or just sensed.

For example, one's speech habits may lead one to explain: "It's not surprising that he did this or that. He's a criminal, after all". In this statement, the "criminal" senses the other person's bias and becomes furious, retorting, "I've done something criminal, and I'm going to serve my sentence, but I'm not a criminal".

"Now I understand how to continue!"

This statement (Wittgenstein, 1953, p. 154) has been chosen because I feel that it is a good philosophical statement, not least as Wittgenstein interprets it in his book *Philosophical Investigations*, from pages 150 to 175. This is the fundamental theme that every human being works with. All the time. Whether we are therapists, scientists, teachers, business leaders, bus drivers, mothers, fathers, etc. The project of life is always to find out how we in this moment will be able to move on to the next moment. With regard to the three parts of the world, we will therefore be able to say it slightly differently, respectively: "Since I know *what it is*, I know how *to* move on", respectively: "Since I know *what it can be*, I know how *to* get on", respectively: "Since *I don't understand, but only sense* what it is, I'll have to *pay close attention to what happens* when I now do what I do". It is our fundamental beliefs that "determine" what we are faced with, what it is and how we can relate to it. And, as I've said many times before, our basic beliefs are "bewitched" and carried by our daily linguistic expressions to ourselves.

To know I've chosen the term "*to know*" as a common term for understanding (grasping with the mind) and sensing (feeling with the body). When you say or sense: "Now I know", meaning has been created. The path to meaning begins the moment you are exposed to something, for example, the impressions in a therapeutic or research conversation.

The act of creating meaning

This act, which comprises several elements, will now be discussed. Each element represents one or more simplifications. The act of creating meaning is in principle an act of simplification. It is an act that, at each stage, reduces a diversity, a potential chaos, to something that is simple enough for you to know how to relate to what you are facing now.

The external context

You should consider whether what you are facing and describing changes with the larger, external social context. People change with the context. The same person behaves one way in war and another way in peace, differently under work pressure than on holiday, differently in periods with enough money compared to periods with too little money. All this is obvious, but many practitioners and researchers choose to ignore this, and may say, for example: "He's a criminal", instead of saying: "During a drunken party he did something criminal".

The immediate context

This is the relationship between the describer and the described. This is also obvious, and should be unnecessary to say, but it must be said for the sake of clarity. A person answers a question based on the relationship they have with the questioner. If the questioner is unclear, and the meaning of the question is unclear, it is natural for the respondent to hesitate when giving the answer. There can often be many answers to the same question, and if the respondent is unsure, she may answer what she thinks will have the least dangerous consequences for herself. Some researchers and practitioners choose to disregard the importance of the immediate context when assessing the answers to their questions or leave the questionnaires with the answer options already prepared for ticking.

Making distinctions

What you face always contains more than one impression. Even the prisoner locked in a soundproof cell in complete darkness receives many impressions. From himself; heartbeat; coughing sounds; the brushing of his hand against his knee; the touch of his tongue on the back of his teeth, etc. In life outside the cell, for example, in moments when other people are also present, there is a diversity of impressions.

Many of the individual elements in each impression are also in motion, for example, light and colours, sounds and silence, smells and touches, handshakes, eyes looking at you, etc. The impressions are there in one moment. In the next, they are replaced by new ones. We *can't* take in all the impressions at once. That would create chaos. We need to separate and focus our attention on some of them. This is called *making distinctions*. With the help of the distinctions, a "picture" is created that provides meaning and not confusion. It is important to remember that such images contain all sensory impressions; they move and smell and taste and make sounds, etc.

When you find yourself focussing on some of the impressions you are currently exposed to, it is also important to remind yourself that you have simultaneously excluded many other possible impressions. You have simplified. We have to in order to avoid chaos. What is it that helps you focus your attention on something and not something else? What is it that determines the actual simplification that takes place? I'll come back to that after the next section.

Putting things into perspective

To make sense of the "picture", it must be set against a background you already know. This allows you to compare it to something you've experienced before and thus recognise what it's about. Usually, the background appears immediately, and the image immediately takes on meaning. For example, the background could be something we've experienced before that pops into our minds, "in our mind's eye". When I say, "There's a mountain over there", I compare the image of the mountain with all the mountains I have hiked over the years and kept images of in my "inner eye".

When you say in each case that it was a big hand, or it was a small hand, or it was a strong hand or a weak hand, it's because you're comparing it to all the thousands of hands you've seen or been touched by before.

If you pass a man standing on the side of the road crying and waving his arms vigorously and grimacing, you might remember the times earlier in life when you met unusual people and say to yourself, He's crazy. "He's crazy". If you just look at the man, and don't turn your head, you might think he's crazy, and perhaps say, "My dear, don't cry!" However, if you turned your head slightly and looked across the road, you would see a car disappearing into the distance with a young person hanging out of the window with arms waving. You might think that the car had something to do with the crying man and ask him, "Did they say anything to you?" The man says that as the car passed, a young man had shouted out of the car window: "You're abusing your fucking cat!" And the man, who is lonely and has the cat as his best friend and does everything he can to ensure its well-being, said he felt deeply offended. After he tells us that it's not so easy to call him "crazy" anymore. We create meaning as an extension of *the way* we have previously created meaning. Some people tend to just look straight ahead, while others have got into the habit of looking around before forming opinions. Otherwise, one creates an image that fits and makes one's perspectives applicable. There's no point in creating an image if you don't have a background to set it against. A lack of perspectives naturally leads to a lack of opinions. It is important to bear in mind that the perspective against which the image is placed is only one of many possible ones. The conclusion reached at is therefore only one of many possible.

The linguistic formulations

These can also be designed differently, as it is possible to have more than one language, for example, expert language or ordinary everyday language. It can be a mathematical language that conveys the impression of certain knowledge, or an everyday language that conveys an understanding that can be applied. It could be a language that conveys an explanation, or a figurative language that conveys something you have sensed but did not fully understand. There are many ways to formulate a description of the same phenomenon. If you accept that expressions have formative power, this becomes an important point.

The language community

If the clinician's or researcher's description is to be presented to a community, it is far from inconceivable that this community will demand and only accept certain distinctions (methods), certain perspectives and certain linguistic formulations. Many other possible descriptions thus automatically disappear.

Are the distinctions and perspectives chosen?

I think they have to do with speech habits and are therefore more or less self-evident. They come from how you talk to yourself and others daily. It's what you constantly hear yourself say that affects your mind in this context. The inner and outer voices "carry with them" both what to look and listen for, and the background against which should be set. I think I've said this many times already. I'm repeating it because I believe it's crucial at times.

A short summary

I've always hoped that those who describe, whether they're practitioners or researchers, could clarify as they write:

- whether they considered the external and immediate context and how it affected the descriptions; or, if they did not take it into account, clarify why
- what distinctions they made, and indicate all those that were excluded
- which perspective(s) they chose, and indicate the perspectives they excluded
- clarify the choice of language used in the wording of the descriptions, and indicate what the consequences would have been if they had instead used the wording that was omitted.

Perhaps readers could also begin to study different texts so that it becomes clear to them what simplifications, the texts represent. My hopes may remain just a dream, but why not dream a little?

Impressions that appeal to reason – and impressions that move – and impressions that do both. Some variations and a little breathing space for the reader

A man goes to a doctor because he has dry skin on his feet. The skin itches, and he scratches until he bleeds. The doctor, who is used to thinking that dry skin is something some people *have*, says to the man, "I'm going to give you an ointment and you'll have to use it for the rest of your life". The man is not satisfied and goes to another doctor who thinks it may have something to do with blood circulation. He therefore asks the man to stand up and bend his ankles. His ankles are quite stiff and can only be bent slightly. The doctor says:

> The fact that the skin on the feet is dry and itchy may be because the circulation is slightly impaired in the feet. And that, in turn, may be because your ankles are a little stiff. I suggest that you get an ointment, but that you also train the mobility in your ankles. Bend your ankles every time you brush your teeth. Maybe one day you can do without the ointment.

She became so nauseous that she threw up. Or: others saw her walking and threw up.

Her body "forced" her out of the situation. The expression vomiting was clear enough, but it was difficult to understand what impression it was connected to. Perhaps we could go back to the time when the nausea started and find out where she was and what she was participating in?

In this context, it may be useful to know that nausea and vomiting occur when the diaphragm changes from being relaxed to being tense, or vice versa, that is, when it changes from being tense to being relaxed. Nausea and vomiting occur during the transitional movement between tension and relaxation. The diaphragm is the large muscle that separates the thoracic cavity from the abdominal cavity and is also the main muscle used for breathing. When the diaphragm is tense and breathing is thus slowed down and becomes less pronounced, emotions are felt less intensely. When you are suddenly frightened, slowing down your breathing can make you feel less frightened. On the other hand, a long "held" (tense) diaphragm may begin to release, and then nausea may occur,, perhaps followed by an outburst of rage, crying or trembling in fear. Or maybe she threw up because she had been infected by a virus or had eaten spoilt food?

He sensed that he had to be quiet, but didn't understand why.

A man sits opposite a woman who is silent and looking down. Her eyes move little. Her shoulders are slumped, and one hand grips the other in a loose grip. This makes a strong impression on him, and he feels a deep sense of compassion for her.

He senses that he should be there and remain silent. He senses that he should sit at a distance rather than too close and feels his way to the right distance. Six weeks later, the woman met the man and thanked him for the way he behaved.

Definition of research

The following definition is inspired by Donald Polkinghorne:

"Research involves the search for knowledge *and the* communication of that knowledge to a community that judges the value of the research in question" (Polkinghorne, 1983, pp. 1–4). This definition could turn any communicated description of treatment into research. Like any definition, the definition above also requires further clarification, namely of the terms: search, knowledge, dissemination and a community that assesses the value.

You can *search* in several ways: talking to yourself or others; reading; writing; shaping using signs other than words (e.g., sounds and colours), etc. We can talk about four types of *knowledge*, all of which can be related to the two verbs: to know and to be able to (act, master). One form of knowing is *rational*, which happens when we grasp or grasp something with our mind. Another form is *practical/technical* and encompasses our repertoire of actions, including expressing ourselves. A third form, which is *relational*, encompasses how we can relate to the other(s) from moment to moment. A fourth form, which is *bodily*, involves sensing one's own body's reactions to what is happening from moment to moment. *Communication* can be of different kinds: speaking, writing, showing in action, etc. The last expression, *a community that assesses the value*, becomes an essential element, especially if this community is to assess the quality of the knowledge. Which community should this be?

One difference between practice and research

I imagine that the process described in the section "The act of creating meaning" is in principle the same for research and practice. But there is one difference. The meaning that is created in treatment primarily has significance within the context of the treatment, that is, for those who are involved at the time the treatment takes place. The meaning created in research is intended to have significance in other contexts and at other times than where and when the research takes place. Meaning created in treatment is thus localised and specific to those participating in it, while meaning created in research is more global and general and is intended for more people than those participating in the research.

Two different researchers

Some clinicians and researchers think that the man crying on the side of the road was crying because something was triggered inside him. They talk a lot about the inner self when they talk about crying people, both to themselves and to others in the language community they belong to. They tend to dig to find out what lies beneath the surface. This is, of course, linked to the fundamental belief that there is something to dig for beneath the surface (von Wright, 1991, p. 94). Steinar Kvale compares such researchers and clinicians to "miners" (Kvale, 1997, pp. 19–21).

One of these researchers decided to travel around Norway to meet all the men crying on the side of the road. Before setting off on his journey, he had made a list of what he wanted to know about the men. In other words, the distinctions had been made in advance. He had chosen the questions in order to be able to compare his findings with previous reports on crying men in other countries. The perspective was thus previous articles in well-respected international journals. Participation was quite good, with 65 per cent of the men willing to take part. Incidentally, this was the same as participation had been in most other countries. From the list, the men were asked how old they were, what kind of education they had received, which municipality they were born in, how much they had earned the previous year and whether they were married and had children, just to name a few questions. They were also asked to tick off answers to 35 questions. When the researcher returned home, the answers to these questions were scored and showed how much depression the individual weeper had. He then collated the entire material and found that the typical crying man on Norwegian roadsides is 42.1 years old, divorced and has 1.43 children, he is unemployed, to name but a few of the findings. The findings were like what had previously been found in other countries and, in fact, very similar to what had been found in Denmark and France. In his scientific article, the researcher discussed the methods and pointed out certain uncertain findings. Since it wasn't easy to know what to do with this new knowledge, he suggested more research with improved methods to explain what the crying man *is really like*. Once you've got a handle on it, you could perhaps create an action programme or maybe even a centre of excellence for the benefit of such men. One of the men got hold of the finished article. He was a little disappointed because it was in English and written so much in mathematical language that he didn't understand it.

Other clinicians and researchers belonging to a different linguistic community regard all oral and written reports as different narratives. The scientific article in the paragraph above is just one of many possible stories about these men. These researchers and clinicians are very interested in the story the individual crying man himself prefers to tell. Steinar Kvale calls them "travellers", and their reports are more like a description of what they pass and experience on their journey. One of these researchers also decided to travel around to meet the men. He hadn't made any plans. He wanted to get to know them first and foremost. He told the men this, and he also said that if he was going to write something about what he learnt, the men should be able to see it and comment on it before he sent it off. When the men realised that they could tell what was important to them, everyone became interested in telling their story. Everyone joined in – one hundred per cent. The researcher heard quite a few gripping stories. He therefore chose to emphasise what seemed important to the men and to highlight what he himself was touched and moved by.

In other words, the distinction emerged of its own accord and was grasped as the stories were told. All the men said they stayed on the side of the road because they were interested in those travelling past. Some of those who travelled past, but far from all, stopped for a chat. What had been good for the men was when they met someone who was kind, polite and generous. The generosity had a lot to do with the passing travellers giving their time and attention. Meeting such people had made many of the men think that there might come a day when they would both stop crying and stop standing on the side of the road. As he wrote down the stories, the researcher became more and more engaged. He went back to the men and discussed whether other Norwegians should get to know the stories and, if so, how. This resulted in two radio programmes and three articles in the colour weekly press. A pop musician became interested and made a song about the men, and this song became quite popular. The researcher, who eventually felt the men were almost his friends, visited them a few years later. Many had retreated from the roadside, and many were laughing instead of crying. The researcher had not quantified how many. Most of the men also said that, after the radio programmes and magazine articles, there had been many more passing travellers who had stopped recently, and they were even kinder, politer and more generous than before.

Some comments

The first researcher comes "from the outside" and is the active questioner (Andersen, 1996). The men are only there to answer. The psychiatrist's standardised interview is another example of the same thing. Jaakko Seikkula, who is inspired by Bakhtin and Vygotsky, calls this a monological conversation; it takes place only from one party's perspective (Seikkula, 1995). One person talks *to* the other. The researcher strives for sobriety and objectivity in their function as an observer.

The other researcher got carried away and was affected by what happened when he met the men. Both parties could ask questions, and both parties could answer. Both "own" and are responsible for the conversation. This is what Seikkula calls dialogical conversations, which means that they are conducted from the perspective of all parties present. They talk *to* each other. What the researcher learns comes "from within" the conversation, namely, from what they create together. The researcher emphasised being a participant.

What is it that makes two researchers, who both meet the same men, choose a position "from the outside" or "from the inside" to find their answers? I imagine that it has to do with the fundamental belief that *either* the nature of the research task requires an expert who can observe, categorise, conclude, explain, predict and generalise, *or* the opposite; namely, that the task requires equal participants who are looking for several ways of understanding and who choose the understanding that seems most applicable and useful. When one becomes either an observer or a participant, it is probably also related to what the basic belief says about "the typical" of what one is facing, crying men on the side of the road.

The same person being researched can appear very differently in these two relationships. When being observed and judged in the "outside relationship", one can easily become insecure, confused and taciturn, while someone participating in the "inside relationship" can easily become calm, thoughtful and articulate.

Based on what I have discussed in this chapter, I believe that the study of human beings is mainly about knowledge of what it can be, and not what it is. What kind of researcher is being moulded when his linguistic expressions are to be mathematical without emotion, and what kind of crying men are being created in the course of the corresponding research process? These are essential questions.

The ongoing linguistic activity in both research and therapy *shapes* all parties: both researcher and researched, both therapist and client/patient. Gareth Morgan makes this question a major topic of discussion in his book (Morgan, 1983, p. 400) (my translation):

> Which people's experiences and perceptions of reality does our research express? Whose interests do they serve? (...) the challenge is to realise that research serves interests and to recognise the human consequences of our research activities. This challenge is particularly relevant at a time when so much emphasis is placed on developing usable (applicable) knowledge, and when many research institutions, funding sources, journals and book publishers favour research with a problem-oriented character. Useful (applicable) for what? Useful for whom? What problem? Which people's problem? These are crucial questions for examining the values and interests that shape the research process.

Marginalise or colonise or prioritise or dominate?

These are big words, but they need to be understood in terms of the diverse and complex process that is the act of creating and formulating opinions. It can be dangerous when someone imagines that they represent superior and "correct" horizons from which they can distinguish between what is correct and what is wrong, whether it is a matter of defining the "essence" of the researched, methods (defining the right distinctions), perspective (pointing out the right theory) or forms of description (choosing the right method of systematisation and formulation). Some people have the courage to believe that they possess this ability to distinguish, for example in certain journal editorial boards and in certain committees that judge applicants who want to enter academia. In fact, there are some people who have this belief in themselves. Some have begun to speak out against this tendency to colonise, dominate and prioritise. Some are selected and included. Some are singled out and excluded.

Sissel Reichelt has questioned the inclusion and exclusion criteria (Reichelt, 1996). She evaluated an academic committee's assessment of two applicants for a professorship in clinical child and adolescent psychiatry. Both applicants, who had many years of experience in clinical practice and had submitted qualitative work for assessment, were not approved for the professorship. The committee described one applicant's work as follows:

> … "could have been presented in a more rigorous scientific manner" … "the empirical material is only used as illustrations and not reported in any systematic way" … "deals with 'this and that' about being a clinical psychologist" … "bears more resemblance to reflections than to research reports" … "(the applicant) lacks a major scientific work, where the ability to systematise in a scientifically rigorous manner is documented".
>
> (Reichelt, 1996)

Any reader will recognise that this means the committee knows what "good" or "correct" research should be. This is not an uncommon starting point for academic committees, and Sissel Reichelt puts it this way:

> Conventional empirical designs, like large parts of academic psychology, are linked to a scientific research tradition. This is based on the notion that true knowledge reflects an objective reality and that it is possible to uncover universal laws. Within psychological research and psychotherapy research, this notion implies that it should ideally be possible to predict and control human behaviour. An implication of this is that practitioners should be able to base their practice on empirically validated experiential methods.

Sissel Reichelt asks about the committee's reasoning for this being the correct basis for the judgement. The committee has not provided an answer, which is a shame. It would have been interesting to know the dilemmas the committee most likely faced, and the difficult discussion it must have had about what research should be and what it can be. It would be valuable for the academic discussion if the committee and other committees discussed a little more what research should or could be (Andersen, 1996a). One book discusses, in an interesting way, how the ongoing, and perhaps not fully appreciated, discussion in academia contributes to standardising the perception of what research should be (Oddli & Kjøs, 1998).

We chose

We chose a form of research that was consistent with our clinical practice. We wanted to be participants, not just observers. We wanted to engage in dialogical conversations instead of monological ones. We wanted to study ourselves first and foremost, based on our fundamental belief that the only person in the world you can change is yourself. We do not believe that it is possible to predict or control other people's behaviour. We have therefore chosen to study the significance of what we ourselves have done with the help of those we have influenced. We wanted to explain where possible; for example, we have explained how many children we met, the marital status of their parents, how many were in foster care, etc.

We have endeavoured to understand what was appropriate, for example, how, from the perspective of certain people, the families fared, or what can cause offence and what does not. But the prerequisite for arriving at much of what we have understood was that we allowed ourselves to be touched and drawn into the conversations with the families and their professional helpers, whether it was in the assessments of the families requested by the authorities or in the research assessments of our own activities that the families were involved in with us. We were therefore not on the outside looking in to gather "objective" knowledge. We were "inside" and, together with those we talked to, obtained the knowledge that will hopefully move the reader out of their own perspective and into that of as many others as possible, while retaining their own, as was the case for us. We wanted it that way. Hopefully, we have also strengthened our ability to sense. What that consists of is difficult to describe because we don't have good words to describe it. Perhaps the quotes in the book will help?

A, for the time being, fundamental belief

If a human centre exists, it is outside the person, between people.

In the community. In the conversations. In the language. In the culture.

It is the encounters between people that are significant for how we live and are shaped. These encounters are constantly changing, just as people themselves move and change.

Life is made up of unstoppable movements.

Part 4

Descriptions from different practices

Chapter 8

Descriptions of collaborating practices with patients, families and networks

The dissolution of the group that had worked together in Tromsø meant that I had to decide how to be organised. After all, I could easily go back to being included in mainstream psychiatry if I just wanted to become an expert again, an expert who was centrally located and to whom people travelled after being referred by, for example, the local doctor. The experiences from the project period in Tromsø were so profound that it was impossible to become a centralised expert again. The experience was that a human problem is best understood and worked on in the context where it belongs. That's why I had to be willing to travel to this context. Moreover, it was often the local helpers who would refer to a specialist. They thought that the patient and/or the family needed something more and better than they could offer, while the people themselves were often satisfied with the locals. Furthermore, the long-lasting and strong relationship that had been established between the local person and the patient and/or family was considered so valuable that it shouldn't be broken.

As a result, I decided not to have my own practice, and the best way to avoid this was not to have any office of my own in Tromsø. So, when someone called and wanted help, I had to say, "since I don't have a room, I'll have to come to you and work with you in your office". Everyone accepted this. If patients called directly, I explained the same thing and said that "if your carer wants to, he or she can call me, and I will come". The local helper organised money if there were travel and/or accommodation expenses. In the years to come, there were quite a few journeys throughout Northern Norway.

When I chose to organise myself in this way, I naturally had to ask myself whether there was anything that spoke against doing it this way. Was there anything that spoke in favour of me not doing it this way? To answer this question, it had to be nuanced according to the different perspectives I was now participating in and committed to. As a university employee, which entailed three perspectives, I was to participate actively in the region's health service, educate medical students and conduct research. The order in which the three activities were listed had always struck me as an expression of their mutual importance. Participating in the health service was most important. Could this way of doing psychiatry be combined with research? Obviously not, if such research required a daily presence in a laboratory

DOI: 10.4324/9781003357742-14

in Tromsø, but nobody claimed that. In a fourth perspective, could such a practice of psychiatry go against the development of the profession itself? This became a difficult question. And what kind of question is this? Is it a political question? Those on the front line were clear in their wishes that this was a form they wanted. The specialists in psychiatry thought the opposite. I chose the first line's view. Perhaps because I originally came from there and had found my professional identity there? If that was the case, what is a professional identity? I didn't realise this last question at the time, and I don't know if I have an answer even today. Maybe this book can find one. Finally, in the fifth perspective, which is personal: can I vouch for such a practice? Yes, both towards colleagues and patients.

The co-operation with the local took a certain form. While we, the local helper and myself, were alone, the first question was: "Is there anything you want me to know before we meet the patient/family, or can we wait until they are here?" It's important that the local could say what he or she couldn't say in the presence of the family, for example, "I'm tired of everything they demand of me", "This is a man I'm terrified of" or "I'm pretty annoyed by the way they treat their daughter". In the beginning, maybe one in four people would say something in private. Now it's one in a hundred. Then we clarified what the local person wanted me to do, either to be passive and listen to the local person talking to the family and then make comments, or to be more active and take the floor and possibly engage the local person in a reflective conversation. It was the latter form that was the most common. Once I became part of such local work, I stayed as long as they, the local professional and the family, wanted my presence. It's remarkable how often just one meeting was enough. Sometimes I came back once or twice, and in a very few cases more than that. In one case, I was there for two years and in another for three years. The tasks could be slightly different. If the local therapist didn't like the patient or the family anymore, my task was to bring out a sympathetic side in them, so that the local therapist wanted to continue working with them. If you brought out the lonely side of the demanding person, it could be easier to work with them, and then it's a matter of looking for openings for a continuation.

There are four questions that can come in handy during a conversation: one I ask only to myself, two I ask openly, and the fourth sometimes openly and sometimes only to myself. The first one, the one I only ask myself, goes like this: "Is there any sign that what's happening now is *too* unusual for the people I'm talking to?" In other words, what is it like for them to participate in this conversation? As well as allowing one ear and one eye to follow *what* we're talking about, it's important to allow the other ear and the other eye to follow *what* it's like to talk. Is the conversation engaging, or is it boring? Is it easy to participate in, or does it become so strenuous that it is more desirable to withdraw from it? It's the flow of the conversation that determines whether it is suitably unusual, not unusual enough or too unusual. It is when it is reasonably unusual that the conversation flows, while it stops when it becomes *too little* unusual or *too* unusual. For example, it may be so unusual that you get scared, don't understand something or are drawn into a topic that makes you feel embarrassed. If the conversation stops, I'll have to find something else to talk about or consider whether we should talk in a different way. Perhaps there are too many of us present? Maybe the "right person" isn't present? Maybe we should meet at their home instead?

The second question is aimed at the interest in participating in the conversation. An opening question could be: "Can anyone tell me how this meeting came about?" or: "Who came up with the idea that we should meet here today?" Anyone present, including the local therapist, can answer. Most often, it has been the therapist who answers first. During the examination of this question, it will become clear who is interested in participating and who is more reserved. It can be useful to find out who organised the meeting, and then hear how the others, who later heard the idea, reacted to it. The important thing about the discussion around this second question is to find out which of them want to talk and which are more reserved and perhaps don't want to talk. This second question came after quite a lot of thought in connection with a "mistake". We once met a family where the problem "was" the behaviour of a little boy. He couldn't sit still and couldn't keep his attention on anything for more than a few seconds at a time. He was pacing back and forth, much to the annoyance of others. The conversation had no flow, but all of us, both the family, who were polite, and we, who tried to be friendly, struggled through the meeting. We all left the meeting feeling uncomfortable, both them and us. My own discomfort was unquestionable, and in the days that followed, I thought a lot about what happened and, not least, what could have been done differently. Then suddenly, the answer came, of course, on a mountain hike, as so often before: what if we could have asked the family, "Who was it that wanted you to come here?" They would probably have replied that it was the doctor. If we had then asked, "What do you think of this proposal?", they would probably have said that they didn't understand it. If we had asked: "If the doctor hadn't suggested that you come here, would you have asked for it yourself?", they would probably have said no. Had we asked: "Did the doctor say what made him want you to come here?", they would probably have replied that he didn't say anything, and they themselves didn't understand what he had in mind. Had we had this little discussion with the family, we might have explained: "Perhaps the best thing would be to call the doctor in the first instance and find out what he wanted from this meeting, and then possibly meet you later if it makes sense".

This second question is closely related to one of two guidelines I try to follow in my work: those who want to talk should be allowed to talk, but what is far, far more important is that those who *don't* want to talk should be let go. The third question is also addressed to everyone, including the therapist: "How would you like to use this meeting?" or something similar: "Do you have any wishes for this meeting?" This seemingly simple question, which took a long time to arrive at, contains many possibilities. Among other things, it is possible to answer: "I'm so tired that I can't think or talk. I'd like to just sit and rest". If this is the answer, you then must work out how best to do this: should she be alone, or should there be someone there; should there be coffee or tea, an ashtray, music or silence? If my starting question is: "What should we talk about today?", I have implicitly mentioned: "Here we will work and not rest!" If my initial question is: "What problem do you want to talk about?", I have implicitly said: "Here we will talk about problems and not successes!" Everyone present gets a chance to answer the question: "How do you want to use this meeting?", and I try to remember their answers verbatim. Occasionally, someone answers: "Nothing in particular", or just "Nothing". They're usually the ones who least want to be there.

When everyone has answered, I go back to the person who answered first and say something like this: "I noticed that you want to talk about (…) (here I try to reproduce exactly what the person said). Can you say anything more?" I talk to him or her for as long as it takes for him or her to tell me what he or she wants me to hear. Then the same with the person who answered number two, then the person who answered number three, etc. So, there are conversations between each of them and me, while everyone else listens. They all get to talk to me undisturbed; if they were to talk among themselves, they would easily interrupt each other before they had finished. In various professional gatherings, the question often arises as to what I do if one of the others interrupts the conversation I'm having with one of them. The strange thing is that when I proceed as described above, there are almost never any interruptions. The very few times it happens, I let the interrupter finish speaking. If I interrupt the person who interrupted, then we're at the same point. When the interrupter has finished, I continue the conversation with the person I'm talking to. If the interrupter, for example, the husband, does this in a very violent way, or interrupts for the second time, I say to the wife I'm talking to, after the husband has finished speaking:

> I have the impression that your husband would like to talk now, while at the same time I understand that there is more you want me to hear. Can I talk to him for a bit now, and then come back to our conversation when he and I have finished?

Everyone who has been asked this question has said, "Yes".

This third question is closely related to the second of two guidelines I have for my work, namely: Those who want to talk should be allowed to talk about what they want to talk about, but it's far, far more important that everyone shouldn't have to talk about what they *don't* want to talk about. On some occasions, the meetings end before you get a chance to sigh, and there is no opportunity for the second or third question. On two such occasions, I can suggest how I talked to myself. On one occasion, we were five men who met, and the image from the conversation was transferred to a television screen in another room where 25 people watched the whole thing. The local doctor was one of the five present. The other three were two brothers and their father. I sat between the brothers, and the father sat between his eldest son and the doctor. The eldest brother immediately took the initiative and showed me a metal box with three tablets; one was yellow, one was white and one was brown. He mostly looked down at the tablets as he talked but occasionally looked up at me, and then he looked me in the eye. He didn't look at the others.

He spoke quickly with a slightly stronger voice than I had when I spoke. What he said sounded something like this: "xxx xxx I xxx xxx anxiety xx x xxx sleep well xxx xxx". He said a lot of words I didn't understand – the x's indicate what I didn't understand. This lasted just over two minutes, and I thought as I sat there: *it's not important that I don't understand. The important thing now is that he finds his form. He'll find it best on his own. It seems like he's scared. Maybe he's afraid of me? What does he know about me? What can I do to make him less afraid? Maybe I should just look at him and not interrupt him. Maybe by looking like this, I can give him the understanding that he can find his form, that is, talk about what he wants in the way he wants. This is not going to work! We most likely won't have a conversation! If it turns out to be impossible, it's important to give up! Don't think about the people watching; they are the least important now! Don't let there be any prestige in this! It's okay to give up! The worst thing would be to push yourself and the others into a conversation that's impossible to have! Let him have a go, but keep a close eye on his brother and father! If they can keep him going, so can I. If they get impatient, I'll try to come up with something. But don't do anything right now. I feel sorry for him. Just look at him as gently as possible!*

Suddenly, he looked at me intensely and spoke a little slower, with a little less force in his voice: "I have schizophrenia. Do you know what it is?" "Yes, I've heard of it", I replied, and he said, "I don't have it a lot. Just a little". The fact that he spoke more slowly, with less power in his voice, made me breathe a sigh of relief and think that it might work after all. I then spoke to the doctor, who said there was a discrepancy between the brothers. He said that it was the younger brother who wanted the meeting and wanted to bring his father as his support. The older brother was there because he had to be, but he didn't like it. The eldest kept trying to say something, but the doctor continued undisturbed. Eventually, the other three joined in, and we spent a long time figuring *out how* to talk to each other. The youngest brother would speak first, then the father, then the oldest brother and then possibly the doctor and me in a reflective way. In the middle of this discussion, the eldest brother asked: "Do you see any signs of illness in me?" I replied that I was so busy figuring out how to talk to him that I hadn't thought about it, and I asked if he wanted me to look for any signs of illness. No, he didn't, and the youngest brother laughed. I asked what he was laughing at, and he said: "He interrupts like that all the time". "What should I do when he interrupts?", I asked, and the youngest said: "You should just stop him". "Maybe he'll be offended if I stop him?", I asked, and the younger one replied: "No, just stop him!" Then I said to the eldest: "If you break into a conversation, how should I stop you? Should I just say stop, or should I put a hand on your arm and say stop?" "No, it doesn't matter how you do it". I repeated my question, and he answered: "Do whatever you want". I repeated my question for the third time and added: "It's important that I do what you want", and he said, "Just say stop". It took us 26 minutes to figure out how to work together. It was well worth it. Over the next hour, the disagreements were clarified, what needed to be different was made clear and what would happen if the difficulties continued was made clear. The elder might have to return to the psychiatric hospital where he had previously stayed for ten years. In the years that followed, the eldest were idiosyncratic in the same way as before, but he stopped *doing* what his brother could not accept, and he has lived in his own house all this time.

Coming back to the situation described earlier, where five women were to meet me: the therapist together with a grandmother, her two daughters and the granddaughter, who is the eldest daughter's daughter. We met the four in the family in the waiting room, where we shook hands and told each other our names. On the way to the counselling room and in the first few minutes in the room, there was a lot of commotion, noise and laughter. The meeting was taking place in an educational institute in another country, and a class of students sat behind a one-way mirror and watched. The eldest of the sisters said as they entered: "Take it easy! Keep an open mind! It's important that everyone is here, especially mum. I didn't dare tell her that there were people behind the one-way mirror, because then she wouldn't have come". The youngest of the sisters said: "I'm just the driver", and she and her fourteen-year-old niece leaned against each other and giggled loudly. The grandmother found a chair furthest from the others, and the situation seemed uncomfortable for her. When she sat down, she complained about the chair and the therapist found a new one.

I thought: *This probably won't work. If it's best to give up, maybe there are other ways? Perhaps the therapist and I could start talking to the oldest of the sisters on our own, and possibly include others as we go along, depending on who is ready for it. Forget the bystanders for now; give up the conversation if it's in the best interests of those who are here! Right now, grandma seems to be the one who doesn't want to talk. Can she be protected in any way?* So, I say to her: "So you didn't realise that others would be following the conversation?" "No, and I didn't really want to come in any case". "Do you think the others would accept it if you just sat and listened without saying anything?" "Yes, I can listen for a bit", she said, and I was able to ask the eldest of the sisters: "Is it okay if mum just sits and listens for a while?" Luckily, it was okay, and now I knew that the therapist and the eldest sister would most likely talk. Her mum didn't want to talk to begin with, and her sister probably wouldn't, but I didn't know what her fourteen-year-old daughter preferred. *So, to myself: leave grandma, the youngest sister and the fourteen-year-old alone for now.*

It has become an overarching discussion in all conversations to first find out how we are going to work together *before* we start collaborating. Attention must be always focused on the collaboration, even *while* collaborating. Perhaps the best way to do this is to let one ear and one eye follow *what is* being collaborated on and to let the other ear and the other eye follow *how* it is being collaborated. The fourth question is this: Who can or should talk to whom about what topic in what way at what time? No human being talks to just anyone about anything at any time in any place. We carefully choose both who and when and where and how. And, not infrequently, it takes a long time to work this out. I imagine that any topic of conversation that arises should be subjected to these questions: Who should be involved, when, how and where.

In the meeting with the five women above, shortly after it became clear that the grandmother could sit and just listen, I decided that I wanted to talk to just the therapist. This happened because there was so much turmoil, and a conversation between the therapist and me could create a certain overview of the possibilities of the conversation and perhaps create some calmness. The other four could reflect on what they heard, if they wanted to. The therapist said that it was particularly her wish that they should gather because she and the others didn't know how to move forward. They were "stuck". She had met the family on and off over the past year and a half. The starting point for the conversations was that the fourteen-year-old daughter was often out of balance. She alternated between crying and rage and had difficulty concentrating on schoolwork. The mother and daughter were usually present, but sometimes the therapist spoke to the daughter alone. Twice, all the four of them present that day had tried to talk to each other. It had failed, and both times the conversations broke down and had to be abandoned. The therapist went on to say that a recurring expression, a "black cloud", had recently emerged, and this black cloud also included the fourteen-year-old's father. It was natural for me to ask, "Is everyone here familiar with the 'black cloud' and is everyone ready to talk about it?" The therapist took a good look around before saying, "Yes, I think so". Then we could talk about it. If she had said she was unsure, I would have said, "If someone wants to talk about the 'black cloud' and someone doesn't, what do we do?" I say we and thereby include myself. I do it because we all, in the moment, have a common problem, namely, how to take the next step.

Harry Goolishian launched the idea that it is the problem that creates the system and not the other way around. The problem creates a system of opinions, and the conversations that arise about these opinions create, develop and organise the community. He said that a problem creates opinions of two kinds: *both* how one can or should understand the problem *and* how one can or should try to solve it. Conversations continue to develop around such opinions. The problematic system is shaped by problematic conversations and/or problematic language. One type of problematic conversation occurs when the people talking together have opinions that *are too similar*. The parties repeat each other and do not stimulate each other to new opinions. Another type of problematic conversation occurs when the speakers have opinions that are *too different*. The opinions are too far apart, the parties do not understand each other and reject each other, and the conversations break down. This is *the big* problem: conversations about a problem come to a standstill. In such cases, the biggest task is to get the conversations going again. This can only happen if the parties become interested in each other's opinions again and avoid having negative opinions about them. Problematic language contains negative descriptions. A description is never negative *in itself* but becomes negative in the ear of the listener. For example, it will easily sound negative, perhaps even offensive, when someone describes another person or their actions as wrong or inadequate. The person referred to in this way will easily avoid participating in the conversation.

A networker or therapist who joins an already established network is well advised to avoid voicing *their* opinions. There are already enough opinions there.

In any case, he or she must avoid having opinions about the opinions that are there. Should this happen, it is safe to say that tensions and scepticism towards him or her will arise. It is safer for the network worker or therapist to instead show interest in the opinions that are there and concentrate on asking questions so that the opinions that are already there can be more easily understood, for everyone in the network. Something that contributes to a problem-solving network is that the members have *reasonably diverse* opinions *and* can talk to each other about them. Reasonably diverse opinions tend to inspire new opinions and ideas. Moreover, the descriptions that emerge in creative networks are formulated in the language preferred by the participants themselves. It is easier to participate in conversations where one's own form of expression is accepted. When Harry Goolishian talked to therapists, he kept saying, "Don't worry so much about what you should do, worry about the few things you shouldn't do!" One of the things you shouldn't do is have negative opinions about other people's opinions. Then you contribute to making the problems even bigger.

Chapter 9

Four practices where language and conversations are central

Uncertainty and perseverance in Western Lapland, Northern Finland

> Only in the exchange between people does a human being become a human being,
> others as well as yourself.
> Being involves engaging in dialogue.
> Where the dialogue stops, everything stops.
>
> Mikhail Bakhtin

Open dialogue in networks

Jaakko Seikkula, a Finnish psychologist, and his colleagues have developed a valuable way of working with the networks that form around psychotic crises. The area they serve consists of six municipalities and 72,000 people, including the towns of Tornio and Kemi. In the early 1980s, a psychiatric nursing home, Keropudas sairaala, was "a place of residence" for 300 chronic, "burnt-out" psychiatric patients. An attempt to transfer those who wanted to return to their home municipalities was largely successful, and the nursing home was able to start functioning as a hospital and receive emergency admissions. The large psychiatric hospital in Rovaniemi was thus completely relieved of such admissions from Western Lapland within a relatively short period of time. What has happened since must be seen in context and as a continuation of earlier movements in Finland. Open dialogue in networks essentially means that treatment must be adapted to the individual patient, and care must be taken not to generalise the treatment of psychotic conditions.

In the early 1980s, they asked families to come to meetings at the hospital in Keropudas when a family member was hospitalised, but only a few families wanted to come. Eventually, they realised that they weren't coming because it was the professionals who decided what the meetings should include and how they should be conducted. After they consulted the families about both what and how the conversations should take place, they began to turn up. These meetings took place in connection with the hospitalisations. When a summary was made, it turned

DOI: 10.4324/9781003357742-15

out that almost half of the first-time psychotic patients who were met in this way did not need hospitalisation. This stimulated major changes in the organisation of the services. The first meetings were eventually organised in people's homes, and not only the other members of the family were involved, but also the entire network that had developed around the psychotic crisis. This required all the staff at Keropudas to be trained to be able to participate in this, and all the staff, around 90 people, received a three-year family-oriented psychotherapy programme. As a result, Western Lapland had the highest density of licensed therapists in Finland. Understanding the importance of addressing such crises as early as possible, they eventually organised six crisis teams in the municipalities to be able to receive enquiries at all hours of the day, all days of the week and all weeks of the year. Anyone could make an enquiry: the psychotic person themselves, their family or friends, other professionals, etc. The member of the team who receives such an enquiry has the task, and indeed the responsibility, of setting up an initial network meeting in the person's home within 24 hours of the call. Usually, this happens within the first 6 hours. The person who receives the call *cannot* refer the task to anyone else but must organise the first meeting themselves.

In each case, a team of usually three people is established to follow the task for as long as necessary. One of these three may come from the outpatient clinic, one may come from the Keropudas hospital and one may come from primary care. This team performs its task regardless of where the patient is, either at home or in the hospital. The team says they are "ready to follow the task for life". If there is a relapse in a case, the same team is re-established as far as possible. The duration of work with psychotic crises varies greatly. It may take just a few days before it's all over or even just one meeting, but more often it takes a long time, for example, two or three years. For the first two to three weeks, there may be daily meetings, later less frequently. Initially, the entire network is often gathered, but later this can be simplified, for example, to individual conversations. Typically, these are open conversations where everyone who is affected and involved in the crisis can take part. Everyone can talk, and everyone can hear what the others are saying. The psychotic person is always present.

Anything that is defined as the network's common problem can be the subject of conversation topics: "What should we talk about?", "Where should we meet?", "Who should be involved?", "Should medication be used?", "Is hospitalisation necessary?", etc. The conversations are conducted until everyone agrees. The psychotic person is present the whole time and talks about what and in the way that suits him or her best. It is not uncommon for him or her to speak in psychotic metaphors that are not so easy for others to understand. The team of three can then talk among themselves to look for meaning in the "meaningless" things the psychotic person expresses. It is not uncommon to find meaning in what initially seemed meaningless through the joint conversation.

The most challenging aspect of this work is to tolerate and endure the uncertainty that is created around psychotic crises. It's all difficult to understand; no one really knows how it will all develop, and everyone feels a great sense of responsibility and wants to become active and intervene. It's not uncommon for strong emotions to play out, which easily increases uncertainty. However, it's the uncertainty that the professionals must try to endure. The most important thing is that the professionals *do not* intervene, summarise or draw premature conclusions. The conversation must be allowed to run freely until agreement on what the next step should be arises naturally.

For many years, the approach has evaluated and researched the benefits of open dialogue in networks. The findings are very encouraging. These findings seen in relation to what constitutes the treatment, namely talking together, have led to important discussions about "what a psychotic crisis is". The research results show that such crises start with real events that frighten the person "affected" by the event. However, the event is difficult to understand because he or she does not have a language for what is happening. Anxiety will thus increase, and meaning is attempted to be created through psychotic metaphors and expressions. When the community gathers and talks about the problem, it can be said that all the words and expressions can help the psychotic. He or she borrows from others' expressions. Together, the community searches for meaning in what initially seemed meaningless, and it is with the help of language that they find meaning and understand the actual event that started it all.

The treatment model described here has been developed gradually through practical, clinical co-operation with approximately one hundred employees in Western Lapland. The new philosophy has evolved through trial and error, with the most important aim being to ensure a safe working community that can withstand the uncertainty of searching for something new. The development process has led to ways of dealing with difficult mental health issues being completely transformed. Instead of controlling patients and their symptoms, the focus is on finding their own resources.

It's not so easy to know in Gällivare, northern Sweden

The network work described here covers four municipalities in the far north of Sweden, where around 60,000 people live. The work, which is aimed at families where the authorities develop doubts about whether the children are getting what they need, is carried out in collaboration between the families, social services and the child and adolescent psychiatric outpatient clinic in Gällivare. The aim of the work is to clarify whether the children are getting what they need or whether they need something more. The clinic's great ambition has always been to reach the children in society who most need to be reached. However, this often involves children whose parents do not dare to ask for help. If they were to ask for help and show their children, they were afraid that someone would take them away. This was a tough dilemma for the clinic. The clinic had strong doubts about whether control (negative change) and treatment (positive change) could be reconciled. However, since their overall goal was to ensure that children got what they needed, they decided to work together with the authorities. The authorities, with the law in hand, can intervene in families' lives.

The outpatient clinic also opted for open conversations. When a child welfare worker calls and asks for help to investigate various issues in a family, they reply that they can come straight away and bring the parents with them. If possible, they also want the person who has reported the family to the authorities to come. Often, it can be a school or pre-school. The latter is often difficult to organise. When the parents and the child welfare worker arrive, all concerns and questions are laid openly on the table in the parents' hearing. It could be that a child arrives at school with few clothes and is hungry, or that a child in kindergarten is very scared and runs away when adults are around, or that someone is afraid of the consequences of child abuse, or that the school is afraid that a child will hurt other children. At this first meeting, parents are also given the opportunity to say whether there is anything they would like to have considered. During this meeting, a plan is drawn up for how the investigations will be carried out. In principle, the parents are involved in planning the examination themselves. The outpatient clinic always has two people present during these meetings, one of whom speaks to the family and the child welfare worker, while the other listens. Every now and then, the two from the outpatient clinic have a reflective conversation between themselves while the parents and the social worker listen. The investigations take different forms from case to case. The network that is included varies from case to case. It is part of the ongoing discussion: who should be involved in what and in what way? Some families are investigated quickly, but most investigations take longer than the four months prescribed by Swedish law. However, it is important that this open investigation work, which always takes place in co-operation and understanding with the child welfare worker, takes the time needed, as this increases the chance that such changes in the families will take place and that the authorities can withdraw their concerns. In most cases, such positive changes in families occur so that the authorities withdraw their concerns. This way of working has also led to an improvement in the relationship between the child welfare services and the families, without the loss of trust that so often occurred before.

All these investigations, which cover all the most difficult cases the authorities can face, have been carried out on an outpatient basis, and the children's relationships with their families have hardly been broken.

As this seemed to be a good way of doing things, it was decided to go back to 20 randomly selected families and their child welfare workers from the first 90 cases to find out what it was like to be involved in this. Before meeting them, however, the investigators from the outpatient clinic went to various organisations in the local community that were familiar with such families and had tried to help them. Schools, health services, hospitals, social services, judges, police and politicians said this:

> We will try to find out what our investigative work has meant to those who have been dragged into it more or less against their will, and try and write about it. If you were to read our report, what would you be interested to know?

Everyone wanted to take part in these conversations, and everyone showed a strong personal commitment. They all had questions they wanted answers to, and they all had a lot on their minds that might make things easier for such families.

What was important in this research project was that the original *investigators* would return to "their" families as *researchers*. The idea was that this would give the investigators the chance to experience first-hand what the investigations had felt like for both the families and the child welfare workers. They wanted the investigators to gain this bodily knowledge in addition to the rational knowledge that research is so often limited to. Bodily knowledge is the knowledge that particularly grips us, shakes us and changes us both as professionals and as fellow human beings. These after-consultations, which the research included, brought a more poignant understanding of the offence caused when parents' ability to care for their children is questioned. This offence, which often comes suddenly, throws parents into chaos that is difficult to orient themselves out of. The importance of language was key; that the conversations were simply conducted in a language that the parents could understand. Overall, it became clear that one of the most important things is to make every effort to get the parents to become participants in the investigations. When the parents became participants and were not left out, good changes usually occurred in the families. In order for them to have a chance of becoming participants, the professionals must proceed slowly. They often have to repeat themselves. They have to speak a language the parents can understand. They need to be very clear about what is going to happen, when it is going to happen and how it is going to happen.

The vast majority, 20 of the 25 children in question, were doing well after the investigation period, two were doing badly and three are uncertain. Three of the children had lost contact with their parents before the child welfare authorities intervened. A further four were taken away from their parents when the authorities intervened but returned to one of the parents during the investigation period.

Conversations with imprisoned men – a research network

Kalmar Prison is one of 13 closed prisons in Sweden. The prison has the highest security routines, and the inmates have long sentences, some of them life sentences, which in Sweden means that they will be incarcerated for the rest of their lives. At the end of the 1980s, the institution wanted to introduce opportunities for the inmates to reflect on their lives and perhaps change as human beings, which in turn might prevent them from reoffending. At the time, Swedish public opinion wanted something to happen in relation to men who had broken the law in relation to violence and sexual abuse. One in four inmates at Kalmar Prison had committed sexual offences. The counselling activities in the prison started in 1989, and Judit Wagner was involved in the work. She introduced reflective counselling. Initially, two guards, one female and one male, talked to the inmates. Critical comments from local psychotherapists that "untrained" people were talking to the inmates led to a change of heart, and a guard together with someone who was somewhat trained in such conversations made up the dialogue team. The team still tried to consist of one woman and one man. These two make up a "normal" reflective team; one talks to the inmate and the other listens, after which the two in the team talk together, while the inmate listens. The inmate decides what the topic of conversation should be; the topics can be related to themselves or to others, to life in prison or life outside, and can be in the past, present or future. Some were interested in talking about their offence, and some were interested in talking about the meetings in court and the sentence, but far from all. In principle, the inmates themselves controlled the conversation.

These practices created reactions among employees, and when it all started, one-third thought these practices were a good idea that should continue and two-thirds thought the opposite. At the time, it was important to organise open meetings for employees where everyone could express their opinions. During these meetings, where strong opinions for and against were expressed, it was very important that those perceived as leaders of the business did not take sides with any of the parties' views, but rather just let them be expressed. This probably contributed to a change in the mood among the employees. All employees accepted that these practices were taking place, and currently, a third of the guards participate as active dialogue partners. In addition to individual conversations, there are also group conversations. An important principle here is that the inmates themselves choose who they want in their group. It is important to be able to trust the others in the group. Even if the groups have one or two staff members, it is also crucial that the inmates decide on the topics they discuss in the group. Initially, these activities were reserved for Swedish inmates, but in open meetings where all inmates could attend, immigrants expressed a strong desire for the same opportunities for them. This has now happened. In addition to the reflective conversations and group discussions, the institution has been keen to develop a conversation culture at all levels of the institution, characterised by openness and mutual respect, both in the corridors and in the prison's workshop and school. Judit Wagner, who is employed as a supervisor for the organisation, avoids meeting the employees taking part in the conversations individually, preferring to meet them together. If one of the employees has something they want to discuss with Judit, they do so in the presence of the others. They can then comment on one another's conversation with Judit as a reflective team.

It was important to find out what these practices had and meant, for better or worse.

Was there anything that was good and can be repeated? Was there anything that should be done differently? Who deserves these answers? Who should get these answers? Who can benefit from getting these answers?

The questions above were written, the meaning of the question immediately arises: what does it mean to know? "Gain knowledge", one might answer, and another might ask, "What is knowledge?" For my part, I imagine that the knowledge produced by research is the same as the descriptions that emerge. And there can be at least three different descriptions. The first type of description includes *what is*. The second type of description includes *what could be*. The descriptions *understand* what it could be within a particular context at a particular time. The third type of description is incomplete and encompasses *what one senses but does not fully understand what is*, and thus cannot be formulated as descriptions in line with the two above. They may resemble this: "This seems to be serious, but I don't understand why", "Here is something that made me feel unwell, but I don't know what it is!", "Here was something that affected me so strongly that it almost hurt, but I don't understand what it was". As a rule, one senses how to deal with this, even if the mind does not grasp what one is facing. The part of reality to which this corresponds surrounds us all the time, and we feel it in our bodies. Some people scoff at such vague descriptions and call them opinions. Others accept this as an important element for all people, including professionals, in their attempts to move forward in life.

In Kalmar, we thought that we should find a form of research in which the significance of the dialogue could be explained, understood and sensed. We also thought that as many people as possible in the network created around Kalmar Prison should have access to this meaning. Fortunately, some in the network wanted to know themselves. The management of the prison wanted to know, as did the Swedish Prison Board in Norrköping. Those in Norrköping were asked to write down the questions they wanted answers to. There were ten comprehensive questions, and all parts of the prison that were in some way involved in the dialogue, management, guards, workshop staff and inmates, were represented when the questions were answered. Naturally, one and the same question yielded many different answers. Knowledge of how *things can be* therefore emerged. Both the questions and the answers were interesting in themselves, but it was particularly important that an exploratory relationship with the prison authority in Norrköping was established.

This provided the opportunity for the next step, namely, to invite various parties to an open, joint meeting. The parties were (1) former inmates who had participated in the dialogue activities but were now either at liberty or transferred to another institution; (2) various people at the prison, such as guards and administrative staff; and (3) "outsiders", for example, from the prison board in Norrköping, from the area's correctional services in freedom and even from the Justice Committee in the Swedish Parliament. Someone from the Norwegian Ministry of Justice also attended one of these debriefings.

One person who chaired the whole thing, in this case, me, began the meeting by calling it a *research meeting* where everyone was together to find out the significance of conversation. Everyone was therefore to be defined as co-researchers. It was also said that the three parties came from three different perspectives, and it was important that the three parties should be able to remain in their perspective in this meeting. It's *very important not to mix perspectives*. The parties could calmly listen to what is being thought and done in the other perspectives and thus compare with and understand what is happening in their own.

The leader of the meeting therefore said that he would first talk to the outsiders about what they wanted to know about the dialogue activity, while the other two parties listened. Then he would talk to the staff while the others listened, and then talk to the former inmates while the others listened. Finally, the whole group would open up, and anyone could talk to anyone. This process is like the one used when therapists examine their own treatment efforts. The "outsiders" could ask questions like: "Is this voluntary, or does everyone have to participate?" "Are there any changes with the men?" "If there are changes with the men, are they deep or are they transient?" "Are there specific topics that are addressed?" "What exactly does this counselling technique consist of?" "What's it like for the staff when one minute they're having a personal conversation with an inmate and the next minute they're raiding his cell?" "What about confidentiality?" "Have you noticed any changes in the institution as a whole?" and so on. There was even one who asked, "Is there any point in having a prison at all?"

The employees commented on the questions they could, and they could also ask questions.

They could explain that this was voluntary and that the inmate chose the topics they wanted to discuss, as well as whether they wanted to hold individual or group conversations. Moreover, they could say: "We used to say 'us and them', but now we just say 'we'" or "Now it's not uncommon for an inmate to ask me for a cup of coffee, which I can offer him on another occasion", or "When you get close to the inmates as people in this way, it makes a strong impression. That's why there can't be too many conversations", or "Now that the former inmates are back, I'd like to know if there was anything we did in the conversations that we should have done differently?" or "If there is something significant in the conversations, what is it?" In the third conversation, the men comment while the outsiders and employees listen. It can be assured that they are listening intently. On one occasion, when four men participated, three of them took the opportunity to tell how the fourth was doing. He was now out in the open. However, it wasn't easy to be there because the loneliness was great. When his loneliness was at its worst, alcohol gave him temporary relief but brought him dangerously close to a new offence. The three men's concern for the fourth made the audience, if possible, even more intense listeners.

On another occasion, when nine men came to the debriefing, one said, "When I came here, I immediately noticed the atmosphere and I eventually dared to talk, and when I was shown trust, I could show trust myself, and then you can talk about everything!" When he heard his own words, he started crying, and the room became very quiet. Another said, "This is not a conversation technique. It's about mutual trust and then you can talk about everything. I myself have been able to talk about what I once did and what I denied in court". Another said, "Such after-meetings are very important for us. It would be good to have more". Another said, "It was good that you wanted to listen to us!" In the end, everything was open, and anyone could talk to anyone. At the end of the meetings, the moderator had said something like this, "On behalf of all of us, I'd like to thank everyone for this joint research, and I wish everyone well wherever they go after the meeting!" But nobody wanted to leave. Everyone stayed and chatted with the person next to them. Everyone was clearly deeply affected and moved. What's more, the outsiders had received the explanations they wanted, and a good number understood more about what these practices could be.

The participatory text

Peggy Penn has recently started her presentations by telling two stories. The first goes back to the mining village where she grew up:

> After a mine was excavated, they were just left as they were, like hidden pockets stuck deep into the ground. After a while they became overgrown and the entrances became invisible. When the children ran and played there, it happened that one of them fell screaming through the invisible entrance. Into the depths. Everyone in the village ran up, in fear and excitement, to see a man being lowered by rope to rescue the child. What I remember most were the cries. Different people from the village shouted down to the child. They waited until they heard a faint crying coming back. When the child was heard, everyone burst into tears and shouted again. But many times, the cries went unanswered because the child died in the fall or drowned in the toxic waters of the mine. In those days, the men who lived there died, then the women. It was as if they all sank into the earth they had dug into. These were my first experiences of the meaning of the voice.

The second was:

> I think my preoccupation with the variations of the voice began before I was five. My mum wanted to be a singer. Usually, our voices have the capacity to assert themselves, announce, break the silence, send back, scream or sing. But they can also hesitate, interrupt themselves, lose their way or stutter as my mother did, while I stood by her side, dumbfounded by her struggle. I remember her hands sweating; opening and closing as if trying to hold on to the words that kept slipping out of them. I knew even then that we were losing our ability to stay together and that I was helpless to stop it. What she couldn't say obviously alluded to the tension that existed between all the members of my family. Our silence consisted of listening carefully and exchanging cautious glances. Perhaps she was sparing us from expressing the emotions we were all afraid of, fear and shame. We all felt safer by not speaking. But I was always afraid that up in this silence, a big accident could happen, and we wouldn't realize it until it was too late. I know that was the beginning of my attempts to reach out for a voice.

The missing voices contribute to our staying away from others, while those we can reveal to others help us connect with them. Incidentally, there is a close connection between our outer, social voices and our inner, private voices. The inner voices "decide" what the outer voices can be, and the outer voices enrich and expand the inner ones. *This needs to be thought about.*

Vygotsky thought that "I am the voices that dwell in me". Peggy Penn points out that "I" can thus become dependent on what the inner voices say. For example, if they say, "Who am I?" it makes me a completely different person than when the inner voices say, "How do I want to interact with others?" or "How do I want others to interact with me?" Penn is particularly interested in how unforeseen and unwanted events affect the balance between the inner voices. Some are suppressed, others are amplified. Some can even become so dominant that the others are completely silenced. It is when the balance between the inner voices is upset that difficulties can arise.

Peggy Penn is concerned with the inner voices that dominate in a negative way, for example, those that accuse oneself or others, those that blame oneself or others and those that hate oneself or others. She realises that it is useless to control or instruct these inner voices. The best thing is to allow a voice that carries the opposite opinion to grow and thereby balance the hitherto dominant voice. She is also concerned about the voices that are missing and which, if they were "heard", would bring more feelings of, for example, protection, security and satisfaction. She has got people to write as part of this work. Whatever topic the inner voice advocates, Peggy Penn suggests that the person write about it, often encouraging this to be done in letter form to a person, either living or dead, with whom the topic formed an important part of the relationship. Writing is certainly not everything. The conversation between her and her clients is still an important part of her work. Two practical examples will hopefully clarify this.

A man in his 40s was bitter and hateful in his relationships with other people. This increased after it was discovered that he was HIV-positive. He had probably been infected through injecting drugs. In addition to using drugs, he also used a lot of alcohol. He explained many of the hardships and difficulties he experienced by saying that his own father had made everything difficult for him. His father was away at work a lot, and when he was finally home, he would get drunk and be absent in that way: "If only my dad had been different, my life would have been different." He was encouraged to write a letter to his late father and come back to the therapist to read it aloud. One can imagine that what happened was this; he transferred his inner dialogue into a written text. He then read the text and thus transferred the written text into an outer dialogue. Part of what he read was this:

> Dad, I've never visited your grave, or sought out your best friend (…) I simply haven't bothered with it (…) *here he pauses a little and continues* (…) but you know what dad (…) *pauses more* (…) writing this letter tonight allows me to say I've missed being able to show love to you (…) I've denied myself that for so long now (…) *at this point he stops and leans forwards, resting his elbows on his knees* (…) *he breathes heavily a few times and starts to cry* (…) *in an attempt to stop the crying he starts to sob instead … his wife, who is sitting next to him and has heard the letter in silence, strokes his shoulder and says "There,*

> *there, it will be alright" (...) he finally straightens up and says:* I have one sentence left, but I don't know if I can get it out (...) I know you tried to do your best (...) until we meet again, your son Bill.

There's a silence as he slowly folds the letter, straightens up and blows his nose. We can all feel that an inner voice of forgiveness has begun to grow.

This letter made such a strong impression on him, his wife and the therapist that he was encouraged to write a return letter, a letter from his father to himself. Peggy Penn emphasises such return letters because they allow a person to experience both perspectives in the relationship. His return letter read something like this:

> Dear son, thank you for the letter you sent! I really liked it! Yes, son, you are right, it is important that a father spends time with his children. Remember, son, that you have the chance to do better than me, and remember you have the chance only once. Yes, I should have sought help, but in the 50s and 60s there were no such mechanisms as therapy. It was completely different times back then. But you're right, I should have got help to talk about my feelings. I loved your mother and my family, as I understand you love your wife and children. They were the most important to me. Until we meet again, we can keep in spiritual contact. Yours ... (father's first and last name)....

His voice breaks as he reads the last sentence, but he doesn't cry. He sighs, then straightens up and shows a big smile. We can all sense that the inner voice of forgiveness has grown stronger. He read the two letters to his mum, and she too was moved by them. She decided to find pictures of her father, and Bill saw pictures he had never seen before. From those pictures, she told stories, and he heard stories he hadn't heard before. His voice of reconciliation was further fuelled. Over time, he became less bitter and less irritable towards other people.

After giving birth to a child a year earlier, a 30-year-old woman began experiencing recurring flashbacks of a rape she had suffered ten years earlier. In this case, as in others, flashbacks meant that the situation was relived as it was experienced at the time. They occurred about once a week and began to affect her daily life. This led to tension and distance from her husband, as well as less energy for her child. In this case, Peggy Penn asked her to recount the rape episode while her husband listened. It had started with her and her (at the time) friend going to a discotheque, and she became loose and happy. He followed her home, and she realised that he wanted more than she wanted to do. He pulled her into a room and tore her apart. *As she told this story, she turned her head the way the man had turned it, and she pulled at her jumper the way the man had done. She spoke quickly.* "I was sure I was going to die, so I gave up fighting to survive". PP: "If someone were to come into the room before the rape was consummated and protect you, who would it be?" She thought about it, pointed to her husband and said it would be him. PP: "What should he (your husband) have said and done?" "He should have grabbed him by the chest and put him up against the wall and screamed, 'what the hell are you doing?' Then he (my husband) should have pulled him out". PP: "Then what would you have done?" "I would have thanked him (my husband). Then I would have hugged him, and then I would have cried". PP: "Maybe you should go home and write down this new story where your husband comes in and protects you, and always carry the new story with you and take it out and read it when the flashback appears?" While she was writing down the new story, there was a tendency for a flashback, but it stopped on its own, and then she didn't have it again.

Chapter 10

Shared context, shared history and shared culture – practices in the North Calotte

The Northern Calotte is actually the parts of Norway, Sweden and Finland that lie north of the Arctic Circle. This means that two of Norway's counties are included, namely Nordland, Troms and Finnmark. In Sweden, it includes one administrative region, the county of Norrbotten, and in Finland one region, Lapland. These five regions account for a large proportion of the total area in these countries. Furthermore, they have a total area of 300,000 km^2. In a European comparison, this is equal to Italy, or the UK plus Ireland. Approximately 1 million people live in the Northern Calotte area today (Groth, 1994). The last glacial period was one of many ice ages that affected the Northern Hemisphere. The northern coast first became ice-free around 20,000 years ago. It is believed that the first humans appeared around 10,000 years ago on this ice-free coastline. They most likely came from the east. Findings from the Stone Age indicate that those who lived in this large area had much in common in terms of living habits.

The area was slowly linked to areas further south in Europe in terms of economy, trade, administration and religion. In the North Calotte, there was a race between the Roman Catholic Church, which built on the legacy of Western Europe, and the Russian Orthodox Church, which represented Novgorod and Moscow in the east. At the same time, the Northern Calotte was a virgin territory, both economically and politically. It was not decided whether Denmark/Norway, Sweden/Finland or Novgorod/Moscow had the right to levy taxes, or later territorial rights in these lands in the north. For centuries this dispute went on, and in the meantime, the population was hard-pressed because two and sometimes three states demanded taxes from the same region.

The term North Calotte is relatively new. It was used for the first time in the late 1950s with the aim of attracting tourists. The Northern Calotte was referred to as a natural region, divided unnaturally by national borders. Many believed that people should behave as if national borders did not exist. The North Calotte consists of three countries: Norway, Sweden and Finland; several languages: Swedish, Finnish Norwegian; several Sami languages and dialects; different ethnic groups and different religious interests. For the most part, the region has lived without conflict. The area is bound together by a web of invisible threads. They share the same experiences and understand each other's situation. They speak the same language, without literally doing so.

DOI: 10.4324/9781003357742-16

In my opinion, there are considerably more unifying factors than dividing lines in the Northern Calotte. People in the North Calotte have the same experience of long distances, both to the capital and within the region. It's just as far from Luleå to Stockholm as it is to the Varanger Peninsula in Northern Norway. People often measure distances in time instead of kilometres. They also have experience of long territorial borders with neighbouring countries, which means many points of contact with each other. No oceans separate them. Only between Sweden and Finland is there water; the Torne-Muonio River, which forms a border. It's no coincidence that the people of Tornedalen don't use the standard Finnish word "joki" for river. Instead, they refer to the border river as "Väylä", which means route. It's a route that binds people together; it connects them and doesn't separate them. The populations share experiences of large uninhabited areas, called the backwoods. The population density per square kilometre is three in the North Calotte. The population also has common experiences from a north-south perspective and a centre-periphery mindset, understood as the relationship between the large population concentrations in the south of each country and the periphery in the north, where they themselves live.

The population has a long collective history in a concrete sense. For almost 700 years, Finland was part of Sweden, as the eastern part of Sweden. Sweden and Norway were in a union for 90 years. For over a hundred years, Finland belonged to the Russian Tsarist Empire. In the Northern Calotte, two of the three countries have belonged to the same nation-state for 800 years. The concept of a national border had no real meaning for the people until the outbreak of the First World War in 1914. They have centuries of experience with cross-border trade. In marketplaces around the North Calotte, people from all corners met. At the important Tornio market, Finns met Norwegians, Sami, Russians, Swedes and Karelians to co-operate in trade. The ancient trade routes crossed the North Calotte and were not stopped by national borders.

The population has shared experiences of major migrations through the ages. Poor harvests in the 18th and 19th centuries forced thousands, especially from Finnish Lapland and Eastern Norrbotten, to emigrate to Northern Norway and its excellent coastal fishing waters. The rationalisation and mechanisation of the timber industry and agriculture after World War II led to a huge wave of depopulation in the Northern Calotte. People moved from the countryside to the city, from inland to the coast and from north to south. Over a period of 30 years, the Northern Calotte lost a total of 170,000 people.

The inhabitants have shared experiences of cross-border religious activity: Laestadian and the established church. They have a common social network. Cross-border marriages and family ties are hundreds of years old. Lifestyles have generally been more holistic; work and leisure often go hand in hand. The population has access to common language bridges in the form of Finnish spoken in Tornedalen as well as in Finnmark. Linguistic understanding has increased interest in literature from neighbouring countries. Books have been translated from Finnish to Swedish and Norwegian and vice versa. There are growing feelings of a common North Calotte identity, which is expressed in shared teaching materials and programmes. A region does not become a region based solely on material interests.

It is cultural cooperation across borders that creates a common identity necessary for deeper cooperation. A former Swedish county governor once said:

> A Middle East could easily be copied to the North Calotte in terms of the different borders, ethnic groups and a wealth of religious, material or spiritual traditions. However, the Northern Calotte is governed by a political culture that brings stability to the region. Today more than ever, the three nations, four languages and five ethnic groups live in peaceful coexistence in the North Calotte. It's a source of satisfaction and confidence, even with a future that is often uncertain.

Our cooperation in the North Calotte

We, therapists from the northern parts of Finland, Sweden and Norway, have similar ways of dealing with and co-operating in human difficulties and crises. We have met and worked together in several different circumstances. Jaakko Seikkula came to Tromsø regularly for many years for the Swedish-Norwegian education programme in Tromsø. I have also taught in the Finnish training programme.

In 1996, we initiated an international network "On the treatment of psychosis" (popularly known as the "Psychosis Network"). Here, more than 30 groups from eight countries, Northwest Russia, Lithuania, Latvia, Estonia, Denmark, Finland, Sweden and Norway, come together once a year to share experiences and consult with each other. Since all groups have responsibilities within defined geographical areas, the annual meetings cover these issues: (1) clinical work and teaching programmes, (2) philosophy: "How do we understand the phenomenon of psychosis?", and (3) research on the results of our clinical work. The network rotates from one country to another each year. After the fall of communism in Russia, we decided to invite two Russians to the "June Seminar" in Björkliden in northern Sweden in 1994. It was the start of a decade-long connection with the Arkhangelsk area in north-west Russia. We travelled there twice a year and worked with Russian therapists in four different locations: two mental hospital wards for adults, one for children and a patient clinic. On 17 April 2002, four of us walked on the river Dvina, still covered in ice. The day was bright with clear skies, warm sunshine and no wind. During the walk, we made handwritten notes about what we do and think in our work, and what we avoid. Here is the list.

Moments for what we do and think

What happens here and now matters – it's here and now that counts

Network meetings

The ideas of networking always follow us: Who is part of this situation? What is each person thinking? What is each person doing? Who is meeting and talking to whom? Who is not talking to whom?

Don't plan before a meeting – don't prepare what to work on or how, nor what the meeting will cover or how it will be handled.

Participants decide when to meet, where to meet and whom to include. It is then decided how to work together *before* the collaboration starts. A step-by-step plan is created according to what happens. Let what happens in the meeting generate the next steps. Problems aren't solved, but they do get solved.

Listen to what participants say, not what they mean

Participants decide what to work on, in what ways and when with whom.

The silence through the listening audience's (the team's) silent witnessing – the answer makes the question.

Just talk to your participants about what they want to talk about.

The patient is the expert on the patient role, and the therapist is the expert on the therapist role.

The focus shifts from individual to network perspective and problems dissolve.

Those who want to talk should be allowed to talk, and those who want to keep quiet should be allowed to remain silent. Participants should be able to talk about what they want to talk about, and *not* talk about what they don't want to talk about.

The team

Language through dialogical conversations.

The philosophy of ethics comes before the philosophy of ontology.

We should consider ourselves an audience, as witnesses, and when we are witnessed, we must ensure silence. Only diagnose if it has a purpose.

The necessary conditions in terms of structures and routines for an organisation to enable networking practices

Appropriate training and education programmes, teams, organisational structures and routines are prerequisites for networking.

Work across the boundaries of professional, educational and institutional backgrounds.

Research must be relevant. What are the outcomes of our work for individuals and families across the region? How can all professionals become generalists, facing and tackling all kinds of difficulties?

Moments for what we avoid doing and thinking

Diagnostic procedures – Medication – Control – The language of pathology – Searching for an "inner core"

Discussions about the patient in her or his absence

Become an expert with cutting-edge expertise
Become a sub-specialist
Individual perspective
Thinking that problems should be solved
Use of questionnaires

Two unpleasant incidents and their impact on work

The first incident was discussed earlier, describing a family with a small, hectic and restless boy who had difficulty concentrating. We worked as hard as we could, but both we and the family left the meeting in discomfort. That feeling stayed with us for a long time, and the idea of overcoming the problem we had obviously hit was shattered on a ski trip in the mountains: "If we had asked the family who had the idea for them to come to us?" They would most likely have said: "Our doctor". If we had asked: "Would you have asked to meet us if the doctor hadn't suggested it?" they would most likely have said: "No". If we had asked: "How come the doctor wanted you to come to us?" They would most likely have said: "We don't know". Then we could have said: "Maybe we should stop here today. We'll call the doctor to see what he wants us to do. If it feels appropriate, we can meet again later".

The second was with a family of four whose daughter was admitted to a psychiatric hospital. She was very upset and, from the first moment of the meeting, she ran between the two rooms that were divided by a one-way mirror. She talked continuously without listening to any of us. Suddenly, she "jumped" on her father and scolded him severely. The father sat paralysed, not knowing how to defend himself against her accusations. In the end, we managed to stop the meeting, but not quickly enough to prevent the humiliation of her father. The experience of how this painful event affected the father and us made us think differently. Some ideas about how we could receive enquiries came out of this, and the first one was: "What is the story of coming here?" In describing this story, other questions became useful: "Who had the idea for this meeting?" To the person who had the idea, if he or she is present: "How did they (the others in the room) respond to your idea?" Or to the others who were present: "How did you react to that idea?" "Did any of you like this idea?" "Are any of you reluctant to come here?" "Would you have asked for this meeting if (…) he or she (…) (not present) had not suggested that you come?" Some of the people who meet us are too eager to start talking right away; others are not. That's why we explored the questions above.

The answers we get help us with our first guideline: "Those who want to talk should have a chance to talk, but what's much more important is that those who don't want to talk should have a chance not to talk". The second guideline was: "How do you want to use this meeting?", and everyone present should have the chance to respond. When the first-person answers, every word must be memorised. Then the same question to the others: "How do you want to use this meeting?" Then memorise each word again, and then the same question – until everyone who wants to answer has answered. Those who are most reserved about meeting often answer: "I have no particular desire". This simple question has proved to be very important, in that it allows for many answers, for example: "I'm so tired that I feel exhausted! I wish I could just sit here and rest for an hour!" If we had asked: "What do you want to talk about?", we would have implicitly said: "We're here to work and not to rest!" If we ask: "What problem do you want to talk about?", we would have implicitly said: "We are here to talk about problems and not about successes!"

The question: "How do you want to use the meeting?", is rich in its possibilities, and it also corresponds well with our second guideline: "Those who want to talk should talk about what they like to talk about". More importantly, they shouldn't talk about what they don't like to talk about.

The conversation in therapeutic meetings

The person who first answered the question, "How would you like to use the meeting?", is asked: "You wanted to talk about this or that (repeat what the person said); can you say more?" or if they could talk more about a particular word or statement they made. The person's answer to that question prompts another question from us. Our questions tend to be network-oriented and often start with who, where, when, how and if. They can be combined with: "what with whom?", "when with whom?", "how with whom?", "who can talk to whom?", "if… with whom?", "who will you be with whom?", etc. Other examples could be: "With whom did you talk?", "With whom do you want to talk?", "With whom can you talk about it?", "Those you can't talk to today, will it be possible one day?", "Can someone help you tell them?", etc. It is very common for those we meet to speak in individual terms. We can often make these relational as network questions. If someone says: "I have a headache", we can ask, "Who knows?" If someone else says, "I'm scared", we can ask, "Have you told anyone", and if they say "no", we can ask: "Who do you want to tell?". When they say who, we can ask: "What would that person say if you told them?" and then ask, "How would we respond to that?"

The question instead of opinions

It was more enjoyable to ask questions, rather than to have opinions about what the participants said. If they wanted our opinions, we gave them. When a family told us what they wanted us to hear, we asked if they wanted to listen to the thoughts of those of us who had listened. Usually, one or more of us had listened to what the families said. To those who will listen, we say:

> When they speak, do what you feel most comfortable with: (1) either listen to them, (2) if you notice your mind going elsewhere, just let it happen! You don't have to listen to them, (3) Or you can just rest or (4) Do something else!

We never indicate what the last one might be, but it allows for leaving the room, interrupting, protesting, etc.

There are different ways to develop what we would call "a reflective conversation" above. Using a one-way window, as we did at first, can be useful during training periods. Now we use it very rarely. We prefer to let everything happen in the same room. Often, two people are sufficient, one talking to the family and the other just listening. Then the two have a reflective conversation about what they've heard. Sometimes there can be three. Sometimes the reflective group can be a full audience of many hundreds. To those who are going to have a reflective talk and are not very experienced, we can say:

> I don't want to instruct you. From previous experience, we've noticed that it's best for the family if you in the reflective group can keep the conversation between you. This means that you talk to each other and are careful not to talk to the family or even look at them while reflecting. If you talk to them or look at them when you speak, they are forced to listen to you and prepare a response. Therefore, they can't let their mind go elsewhere if it feels natural.

Essential elements of reflective conversations

What we now explicitly recommend, but do not instruct, is: "Think about what you heard, and not about what you didn't hear, e.g. what you think about what you heard!" We also encourage the reflectors to first summarise what they heard and then reflect on it in a questioning way. We also encourage them to be careful with opinions or meanings, which can easily sound like "you should" or "you shouldn't", or even worse: "You should instead of what you thought or did". This can easily make the participant or family feel that what they thought or did was not good enough.

Looking back, we can see that the various changes in our practice came about through our own practice, or perhaps better to say, in response to our poor practice. These practice changes made the treatment process more comfortable, or perhaps better to say, less uncomfortable for us. Initially, we strongly thought that the theories of practice (therapy) should influence our practice, and we prioritised the theories before practice. Perhaps the general knowledge of the theories made them attractive? Perhaps our affiliation with the university made us think that we should value theories before practice, as is common in academia? We decided that theory should be "descriptions and understandings" of what our practice consisted of, and we searched for the typical and general in that practice. However, to make descriptions, we had to find an appropriate language, and to understand we thought we first had to "understand how we understood". The understanding of the process of understanding we called "epistemology" – how knowledge can be developed systematically. We also believed that we had an internal way of grasping reality, and we also believed that we had to change our way of grasping according to the new relational view of knowledge. It was common at the time to say that we needed to "change our lenses". Our interest in developing our view of knowledge came not from ourselves but from the international field of family therapy. We were inspired by three views of knowledge: first Gregory Bateson, then constructivism and finally social constructionism.

What was useful for our descriptions and understanding of practical situations were certain concepts and formulations. Bateson went "one level up" to understand his way of understanding. He believed that it was useful to clarify the assumptions of one's understanding, one could also say the basic assumptions that affect one's understanding. In his somewhat ironic chapter in *Mind and Nature* called "What every schoolboy knows", he mentions the basic assumptions with examples: (1) science strengthens or weakens assumptions (hypotheses) but doesn't prove anything, (2) the description and what is described are not the same, (3) all experience is subjective, and we create the image we readily believe we get. The process of creating an image or meaning passes us by unnoticed; the product, namely, the image or meaning, is what we become aware of, (4) to perceive and understand reality, we must cut it into pieces and separate them, but that is not necessarily the right way to separate, (5) Language simplifies and emphasises that something has properties. It would be better to make it clear that, through the description, something is "shaped", (6) a person's two eyes give different versions (images) of the same reality they are looking at. The two versions, when blended into one image, make us see depth: something comes closer, and something becomes more distant. One of the two eyes sees independently, becoming a perspective for the other eye. Similarly, when two ears hear the same sound slightly differently, one can hear where the sound is coming from and turn to see what it is coming from and (7) within linear relationships, something is transformed from one part to another without anything returning to the first. Such relationships exist in the Pleroma, the non-living part of reality. In circular relationships, there is a mutual influence between the two parts. When one part interacts with another, the second part reacts back to the first. Such circular relationships are found in Creatura, the living part of reality. All the above are relationships.

Bateson's definition of mind was fascinating but not necessarily easy to understand: a chain of interconnected elements that mutually influence each other through a circular motion. This means that a person becomes part of their consciousness and, at the same time, part of other parts of the circle, such as people and nature. The person can influence other parts of the circle, and the circle as a whole becomes the context that gives the person both opportunities and limitations for what and how they can influence their surroundings and themselves. What creates life, a flow or communication in the circle is the influence from one part to another. The influence from the first part is somewhat different from that of the second part. This represents a difference that Bateson called an "idea". A conversation between two people can be an example of a circular movement; the connections in the body and the flow of information through different organs can be another. It is linked to a change occurring when a "difference makes a difference". Such circular motion becomes recognisable when the flow through it follows a certain type of pattern. For example, the information contained in the genes induces a pattern, such as two moving arms and two moving legs, etc. There are some basic "ideas" or governing rules for patterns that connect. This was a crucial line of reasoning for Bateson. But to what extent did we understand it? And to what extent was it necessary to understand it to do practical, relational work?

A circular movement can be connected to other circular movements: one person to another person, to society and to nature. The different patterns are different. When something in the Pleroma is brought out of balance, homeostatic processes are provoked. Everyone is tempted to be brought back to what it was, or at least to an acceptable balance. The thermostat was used as a metaphor to illustrate this point. For example, if one part of a society introduces a new and unusual way of living, tensions in that society may increase. If the rules of that society are not sufficient to bring balance between the old and the new, a group may break away and establish a new and different society. Bateson called this process schizogenesis.

This reasoning inspired the term "double bind" as a way of characterising specific events in a particular relationship. The relationship might be that a son lives strongly attached to his mother. He seems to be dependent on her and he cannot leave the relationship. Specific events may occur where the mother says, "You're so good!" but the way she says it contradicts what she says. He understands her way of expressing herself as: "You're nothing! You don't do anything!" How can he handle this situation? Since he can't withdraw from his relationship with her, he must receive and accept the two conflicting sides of what she says and expresses. He can't favour one side of what she says over the other. Therefore, acting like "a crazy person" with no comprehensible meaning can be a solution. The "double bind" theory had negative effects on practical work under certain circumstances. Some took these ideas literally and referred to the mothers of "schizophrenic" people as "schizophrenogenic" mothers; in other words, mothers who produced "schizophrenic" children. At the same time, the theory aroused great theoretical interest in human relationships and communication between people. Eventually, we dared to ask questions like, "How was what we understood from Bateson's writings useful for our therapeutic practice?" We realised that we became part of a system when we started working with the system. It stimulated us to describe and understand how we ourselves were connected to the system, both for better and for worse.

Different approaches in reflective conversations

In retrospect, we can see different approaches in our work with reflective conversations. We have to admit that it took a while before we were able to reflect, because we often thought: "How will what I'm saying work?" and "How should I speak for it to be useful?" It took a while for us to forget about the impact of the words on the listeners. Later, we referred to what we said as "hidden" instructive reflections. They could be like this: "If the father becomes more decisive, what will happen?" "If they decide to connect with the grandmother, what would it be like for her?" We had to constantly remind ourselves that our reflections were just something we were offering, something that could be used or just pass by those listening. In a new period, we tended to use our own metaphors. Two examples will hopefully illustrate this.

One was a conversation with a couple where the wife was looking for a new language. As it turned out, it wasn't just her, their two daughters were also looking for a new language. The language should fit their desire for freedom and reaching out. The three women seemed to be looking for a new lifestyle. Literally, they were often away from home. The man, who preferred to continue the quiet life he had before, was very concerned about what might happen to them. Could they find something interesting that would make them leave him? He was very worried. Our reflection was like this:

> When I heard what they said, I got an image of someone going away to collect flowers. From time to time, they came back with beautiful flowers. Someone at home received the flowers and made a beautiful bouquet of them. Someone was searching and someone was holding and protecting what they found.

The second example is also about a couple who had different interests. One was influenced by Eastern mythical ideas, the other by more Western pragmatic ideas. The conversation with them was about differences, some of which were so great that the relationship was at risk. Our reflection was like this: When I listened, I imagined a sky where there were two smiling suns, one coming from the east and one from the west. It was as if they were saying 'let come, let go'.

Such reflections using metaphors disappeared. Most likely because it felt uncomfortable to make ourselves so central. We developed an understanding and a feeling that we should do as little as possible at the meetings. The less central we were, the more central those we met could become. From then on, our ambition was to stay within the metaphors of those we met.

Practical examples of different approaches in reflective conversations

All in one room

At first, we used one-way mirrors and changed the sound and lighting. After a few months, we switched rooms to make it more even. The family and the therapist went behind the mirror to listen to the reflective group in front. After the reflections, they switched rooms again. A few years later, we stopped using one-way mirrors and let everything take place in the same room. This required encouragement to the less experienced members of the team:

> We encourage you to have reflective conversations amongst yourselves. That means you don't talk to the family and even don't look at them when you're reflecting. If they're being looked at or talked to, they have to work out a response and can't let their mind go.

Two professionals

One of the two talks to the clients/family, while the other just listens. One asks the family/clients if they want to hear what the two professionals thought about the first conversation. If they agree, the two can reflect on what they have heard while the family/clients listen. Then the family/clients respond.

A therapist

When there is no team in the room, the individual therapist can reflect alone. After talking with the clients/family for a while, the professional can say, "From the conversation we've had, some thoughts have come to me. Would you be interested in hearing them?" Since the ideas were generated from the conversation between them, they must be formulated that way. When reflecting, the professional discreetly looks down or to the side to allow the clients/family to more easily decide whether to listen or let their thoughts go. We need to constantly remind ourselves that our reflections are just something we offer. They may be used, or they may just pass for those who are listening.

A network reflects

The individual therapist talks to someone in the group or family while the others listen. After a while, the therapist can ask the others if they would like to share what they were thinking. When this happens, the person who spoke first listens and then responds to what was said.

A group therapy reflects

The individual therapist can talk to one member of the group for a long time and then let the others reflect or talk to each other for a shorter time, and after each short conversation, let the others reflect.

Staff meetings and group counselling

One person leads the meeting and talks to one or more people who are engaged with a particular client/patient. The rest of the staff listen first and then reflect. If the client/patient is present, at the end of the meeting, she or he can comment to the person who has led the meeting.

Live consultations at conferences where the audience reflects

One of us talks to a family and their local therapist in front of an audience. An example: One family told us that their son would often act out, and they waited for it to stop. However, the episodes were demanding and the parents hoped that it would stop one day. They also said they didn't understand him because he didn't speak, he just acted out. When the family and the therapist had said what they wanted to say, they were asked if they wanted to hear what the audience had thought. If they did, one of us encouraged them to listen or let their thoughts go or rest or do something else. One of us moved away from the family and the therapist and towards the audience, encouraging the audience to talk to him and not to the family. Someone in the audience gave their reflections: "Parents should be firmer!" That person was asked: "It sounds like you had an opinion. Can you accept the word opinion?" Since one of us thinks that an opinion could easily sound like an implicit criticism, I ask: "How do you think what you said was for the family to hear?" If the participant says "maybe it's difficult", one of us can ask: "If you were to express the same opinion in words that were easier to hear, what might those words be?" If the participant can't find such words, one of us can say that he has some words. If it is accepted, he can say: We all heard that the episodes of acting out are troublesome for everyone. If they found meaning in the boys' behaviour, would that help them to stop him? How could they search for meaning? With whom?

Reflective meeting with authorities present

The habilitation services in a city in Sweden are very network-oriented in their thinking and practices. They deal with all kinds of functional variations, both congenital and those acquired through accident or disease. Staff from the service, together with members of natural and professional networks and one of us, met to shed light on the situations of people with functional variations from different perspectives. The meeting was transmitted live on TV to a neighbouring room, where others from the services, along with others and different authorities, watched. The meeting focused on a woman with mental health difficulties who was the mother of a four-year-old boy. She was in her late 20s. Five people from her professional network attended. Many concerns had been raised about the woman's motherhood. She was divorced from her son's father, who had greater mental health difficulties than she did. She had her own natural network, but the professional network was currently more useful. She was constantly afraid of losing her son. She was especially afraid that the neighbours, whom she had noticed were paying close attention to the way she dealt with the boy. She felt that she couldn't make a mistake and was afraid that it might happen. We realised at the meeting how the different people in the professional network helped in different circumstances. Each of them engaged in different issues that did not overlap. One of her own concerns was how her son could be told stories, as she could not read herself. At the end of the meeting, they were all asked if they wanted to move to the next room to listen to what the audience had thought. That's what happened. Among those present in that room were the heads of school services, social services, the public job centre and others. They first shared their thoughts. Then they started asking the mum if she could give advice on what they could do to help others in her situation. She stated her practical advice very clearly, and most of us thought: Who can best supervise whom, for example, in the field of people with "functional variations?"

The second example was a national Norwegian conference on coercion and voluntariness in mental health care in Norway. The conference was the result of collaboration between the organisation of relatives of psychiatric patients, the organisation of psychiatric patients in Norway, representatives from the professional organisations of Norwegian psychologists, psychiatrists and mental health workers and the University of Tromsø. The conference and its participants were determined to be experiential and experience-based in a certain way. The first five people, two mental health workers, a psychiatrist, a psychologist and a police officer, spoke about their experiences of restricting people using force. Many in the audience of 350 were patients and relatives. In addition, mental health professionals, mental health educators and researchers, as well as mental health service administrators participated. Next, three relatives spoke about their experiences while everyone else listened. Then three patients spoke about their experiences, and everyone else listened.

At the end, five people from the Norwegian civil services took to the stage: the chief of police, someone from the top level of the health administration, a chief administrator from one of the five Norwegian regions, someone from the board of the Norwegian Psychological Association and someone from the board of the Norwegian Psychiatric Association. They were asked: "What has this conference done to you?" They willingly gave their spontaneous, rational and emotional answers.

Increased awareness of expression

The new "reflective modes" made us more listeners and less talkers, and we paid more attention to how people expressed themselves. We noticed that people would start talking, then stop and start again, maybe stopping a second time and starting a third time. This transcript illustrates exactly that:

> I want to (…) ask for (…) uhm (…) when I was finally sick, my sister called my mum and said: you have to come back there, you have to come to see Mary. And my mum came back. And (…) and I didn't like it very much, because then my father had left again. It was very (…) it was terrible. You know (…) I almost got the feeling that (…) I caused (…) I caused (…) I was in my own crisis, but I also caused people around me their crises. It was like a chain reaction: something bad happens here, then something else goes by. Something quite terrible. You know that everyone has a small share of it. I don't know how anyone else would deal with it (…) uhm (…) (…) I mean in an ideal situation (…) I don't know (…) I mean (…) in an ideal situation I guess I wouldn't be sick (…) in an ideal situation I guess (…) actually I don't know what would happen in an ideal situation how I would react to it (…) if, if, (…) to be someone if (…).

Such events taught us that speaking is searching through one's words to find the best ones to express what is felt in the moment. And we, as listeners, should be very attentive and very quiet and absolutely must not interrupt this search. Just be witness(es) to it. New questions related to the spoken words became part of our repertoire. At the same time, we realised that the questions had been asked three years earlier without us noticing their use. On an earlier tape, we could hear and see a meeting between an elderly couple, a local therapist and one of us. The therapist didn't know whether to "give them advice or be with them where they were". The couple had two daughters: one was diagnosed with schizophrenia and wanted to die; the other was severely affected by anorexia, and everyone was afraid she would die. The father was concerned about what would happen after his parents died: "Maybe they'll commit suicide", he said in fear, when his mother tried to comfort him by saying: "God, the big boss, will help them". The therapist said one word had been repeated many times lately: "tsores". She asked about the meaning of the word. "Problem", the mum said. "No, it's bigger", said the therapist, "grief (…) pain (…) both grief and pain", and silence filled the room. The therapist was asked: "What kind of grief is it?" (…) long pause (…) "Is it the kind of grief you have alone, or is it the kind of grief you have with others?" (…) When the therapist's voice cracked faintly, she said: "Together with others", and seriousness crept into the room. "And the pain part (…) is the pain in the heart or in the mind" (…) "the heart" (…) "What kind of pain is that?" (…) after a long pause: "The pain you feel when you reach for something without reaching it".

Mary, who had been ill and trying to look after herself (T is one of us and M: is Mary). T:

> How do they (…) in your family (…) see you? Do they see you as a person who should never ask for anything (…) or do they see you as a person who deserves to ask for something for yourself (…) How do they see you?.

M:

> I'm not sure (…) I (…) uhm (…) I don't think they see from that… I think that (…) you know (…) looking at (…) I guess the family I grew up in (…) we were supposed to be self-reliant (…) independent was the big word in my family.

T: "Self-reliant?" M: "What (…)?". T: "Independent?" M: (nodding) "Yes. Independence was the big word in my family (…) And (…) You know I feel like I got the message there". T: "I'm sorry, you feel that (…)". M:

> I feel like I got that message there (…) right (…) and I feel like that was something that I really incorporated into my life (…) I've (…) no (…) as soon as they weren't responsible for me it became (…) it wasn't an issue anymore, I mean they don't talk about it anymore, you know (…).

T: "(…) (…) but it's still there…".

The word independent had been mentioned twice, and as she said and heard the word, her voice dropped, and a sad look came over her face. It was as if she was struck and touched by the word. One of us decided to investigate that word but had to wait since she wanted to say something first (what was transcribed above).

T: "How was the word independent expressed? Was it in the open, or was it implicit? Or (…)? How was it expressed?" M: "Well… it was verbal" T: "Verbally? The word independent?" M: "Yes". T: "In the sense of being independent or independence in general, or (…)?" M: "We should be independent. They wanted us to be independent (…) and (…)". T: "So how (…) when you got to know the word and let that word become part of yourself (…) what do you see in that word if you look at the word independent?" M: "I don't like it. I personally don't like this word very much. Partially (…)". T: "Do you see things that (…) says more, what don't you like when you look into the word, or look at the word?". M:

> Well, I see (she starts to cry) (…) talking about loneliness is so hard for me (…) you know I just (…) this was something I was trying not to think too much about (…) uhm (….) I guess the word independent means to be alone (…) and for me it gets lonely (…) to be alone (…) uhm (…) that was the word (…) we used to talk about being independent and I finally said: don't use that word about me anymore. It reinforces something that I really don't like. Had to do everything myself. Had to (…) I've always felt like it's been forced on me (…) for me (…). What I want to do is just (…). I don't think independence is a virtue. I don't believe that at all. I mean being alone (…) uhm (…).

(She (…) is slightly bent forward as if she is collapsing and one hand is holding the other hand).

> Had to deal with things myself (…) uhm (…). I just don't (…). I don't (…) I don't think I treat other people like that (…), but I treat myself like that (…) I feel like I treat other people like (…). I try to give support at least when I can (…). As for me I (…), it's like I don't seek support (…) instead of (…) maybe I do (…). I think about a year ago I finally realised that independence was for me (…) (…). I used it all the time to describe me and finally (…). I'm not independent, no I'm not independent like you think I am (…). I may have grown up with the idea that I should be, but that's not what I believe in now.

(She stretches her back and moves her hands to her sides and opens the upper part of her body again).

> I believe that people should be supportive (…) believe in being co-operative. You know be strong all the time. So that it's something that I feel like I (…) it's valuable for me to come here and talk about things that I don't want to talk about.

T: "If your mum were to look at the word independent, what would she see?".

M: "She wanted to see strength...". T: "And dad?" M: "Also strength (she stopped for a while and laughed) (...) it was interesting, because he wants to see a different kind of strength than my mum (...)". T: "And your sister?" M: "She will see what I see".

Two questions above were important: (1) How was it (the word independent) expressed? and (2) In the way you should be independent or independence in general, or (...)? The way she answered indicated that she could stick to the word. Her answers to the two questions told us that she was ready to explore the word. If she had answered the questions with some form of disgust: "That word destroys me" or "I hate that word". It would probably not have been possible to investigate the word. An example in the following indicates when words should just be let go. But before that, a sketch of the speaking process:

Insert two people talking

One person speak the other person listens. The listener not only listens to each word but also sees how the speaker receives their own words. The listener notices that some of the speaker's spoken words are not only received and heard but also move the speaker. These movements of the speaker can be seen or/and heard. Sometimes a shadow crosses the speaker's face, their hands may close or open, there is a cough, a tear may appear, the person pauses, etc. The listener realises that the spoken words have a meaning that makes the speaker relive something she has experienced before, without the listener understanding what it is. The listener is not infrequently carried away and moved by noticing that the speaker is moved. Those moments when both are moved are good for launching a question or comment, which in turn keeps the speaker's movement and the joint movement going.

Here's an example of a "too strong" word that wasn't researched. A therapist wanted to do a consultation in front of an audience. He explained that the day before, he had been called to the prison because one of his clients had been taken there. The client's mother had been terminally ill and asked her daughter, the client, to end her life. She did so and then called the police. The therapist said that he had been in the same situation two years earlier, when his terminally ill father had asked the same thing. He cried and said he had been unable to fulfil his father's wishes. In the middle of his crying, he said the word "suffer". The word hit him so hard that he sobbed convulsively. One of us, who was speaking to him, decided not to touch this word. Instead, the person asked about another expression he had used just before: "I don't want to burden others". It gave him a chance to leave himself for a while and focus on another person: "Which other is it important not to burden?"

Expressions without words

Laughing, crawling and hitting are examples of wordless expressions. Two situations described below indicate how such expressions can be handled.

Smiles/laughs

Present at the meeting were a thirteen-year-old girl, her mother and aunt, her mother's mother (the girl's grandmother (GM)), the local therapist (P) and one of us (T).

The therapist had met them over the past year. The reason they came to her was the thirteen-year-old girl, who was unbalanced. She cries and acts out and has difficulty concentrating at school. P wanted one of us to be present because she and her family didn't know how to proceed with the therapy. For the most part, the girl and her mum had come to the therapist, sometimes the girl alone. The four of them had tried to get together, but both meetings broke down. From the very first moment, there was a lot of noise and movement. A special laughter filled the room, and the thirteen-year-old and her aunt laughed the most. In order not to be annoyed by it, because it can easily disturb listening and distance the participants, one of us reminded them that laughter could be the only way they could express themselves in this moment, in this context. If T stopped the laughter, how could they be present?

But when the noise made it very difficult to hear, one of us told the therapist:

T:

> That's one thing I've noticed when we've been talking (…) there's been a bit of laughter in the room (…) even though the issues we've been talking about have been very serious (…) and I've been thinking all the time (…) if laughter could talk what would the words be (…) do you have any ideas of what those words would be?.

P: "I've thought about it a lot (…) I've been very aware of it (…)". T: (…) "Are they happy words or sad words?" P (without hesitation): "No, they are sad (…) I think they are really (…) uncomfortable (…) so uncomfortable to talk about this kind of (…) very sad (…)". T: "You feel uncomfortable (…)". P: "No, I think the laughter will really say (…)". T: "Is it so uncomfortable that we should avoid talking about it?" P: "I don't know (…) I think different people in this room have different feelings about it (…) and again I'm protecting (the granddaughter) (…) because I think she laughs the most". T: (…) "I feel very insecure (…) if the laughter had words and the words were too sad to talk about (…) how could we proceed then?" P: "I don't know (…) it could be a dead end (…) it could be that (…) that could be what I'm asking (…)". T: "Do you feel that everyone wants to talk about these sad things?" P: "I see my grandmother shaking her head". (The grandmother is now moving on the chair as if she wants to talk, but one of us continues to wonder.) T: "That's another question (…) if there's anyone who doesn't want to talk about it (…) (the grandmother clearly wants to talk, and she is let in) (…)". GM:

> We're here to talk about it (…) if we can't talk about it (…) how to get it out and sort it all out and try to deal with it. (…) we have to talk about it (…) some people are uncomfortable (…) so am I (…) I haven't been through this (…) it's

> not very easy for me to talk (…) we can't put it under the carpet to protect my granddaughter (…) we can't sort it out unless we talk freely (…) she's only thirteen (…).

(Looking at the granddaughter.) "I had a lot to deal with when I was your age (…) I didn't have anyone to go to either (…) If you can't get it out in the open, how can you deal with it then (…)?" GM tells us that she has cancer, the same type that her closest boyfriend has. They are on the same medication, and her friend is dying. They all know it, but for various reasons, they haven't been able to talk about it. The reason the two previous meetings broke down was that her grandmother had been so angry when she realised she was dependent on other people.

Crabbing and beating

A six-year-old boy, his mother and father, the local therapist, a translator and one of (…) us were present at the meeting. The mother had revealed a year ago that the father had behaved promiscuously in front of his son. In the first part of the meeting, the father spoke eagerly about how the situation at home was better now. He was sweating profusely as he spoke. His wife took a handkerchief from her handbag, which the boy grabbed and took over to his father to wipe his forehead. The boy then went back to his chair but couldn't sit still. Instead, he bent down on the floor and crawled noisily under the chairs the rest of us were sitting on. The noise affected the conversation his father and one of us were having, but the words of the conversation could still be heard. When he passed his mum's chair, she spoke to him, and he answered her. One of us therefore said:

> We have two conversations going on at the same time (…) and that may be ok (…) but should we take one at a time (…) we can imagine that the boy's crawling here is his way of participating in the meeting (…) if we think that his crawling body could speak, what would the words be?.

The mum became thoughtful and said: "I have to think". The father said: "He wants attention", and one of us said: "No, not him. What would his crawling body say if it could talk?" After searching for words for a while, the father said: "Give me attention!" "And who are these words addressed to?" The father: "To me". "And how would you answer that right now?"

The mother interrupted and said that the boy wants his father's attention at home when he does his schoolwork: "But my husband gets annoyed easily, and when he gets annoyed, he hits the boy". To the father: "So you hit him too?" "Yes, sometimes". "How do you hit him?" "When he makes noise". "No, no. How do you hit him?" "I hit him". "How do you hit him?" "I hit him". "Do you use your hand?" "Yes". "Which hand?" He raised his right hand. "Do you hit him with an open hand or a closed fist?" "I don't know". "What do you think you're doing?" "I don't know". One of us turned to the boy, who was very restless now, and knelt on the floor. "When your dad hits you, does he hit you with an open or closed fist?" At this moment, the boy raised his voice and shouted: "I can defend myself more now". "Does he hit with an open or closed fist?" "He hits with his closed hand and pushes with his open hand". In a very loud voice, he said: "I don't care". (One of us said in his inner voice: "But I care!") and asked: "What hurts more, the closed hand or the open hand?" "The closed hand". Then one of us turned to his father, raised his closed fist and asked: "If your hand kept hitting your son, stopped and could talk what would that say?" The father was confused and so was the translator, so everything was repeated and the father answered after the question was repeated a few times: "Peter, stop what you are doing, because what you are doing is wrong". He was then asked how he would say it, and after a long time, after having the question repeated four times, the father said: "I will say it calmly, slowly and firmly".

Feelings within feelings

The therapist and a separated couple were present. The husband wanted the separation; his wife did not. She just wanted him to come back as a changed and better man to be with. The tension in the room was high, and when he spoke, she wrote down every word he said. Since they were expressing very specific descriptions of each other, and talking about these descriptions seemed to reinforce each other, one of us turned our attention to their seven-year-old son's perspective. The father's (F) parents had divorced when he was seven. The father and mother have their son (Peter) at different times. When he was with his mother (M), he often expressed himself with anger. At home with his father, he cried. His father thinks he cries because he feels torn between his parents and therefore gets very angry when he is with his mother.

F:

> Peter asks me; why do I feel scared at my mum's when I'm not scared here? So, it often seems like he feels afraid of mum, and when he's at my house he's more sad (…) less afraid. The places I see him in and I hear him in and the places his mum describes him in are not the places I want my son to be. I want him to be in a world he can trust more. It's very sad that (…) to see my son in the kind of world I grew up in. Where you spend all your time paying attention to what's going on around you and not paying enough attention to yourself.

(…)

T: "Did it happen early in your life?". F:

> Yes. It was chaos (…). I didn't feel that all the people were spending time with me. There were so many strong emotions flying all over the place. It just (…) the feeling of being in a safe centre of things really wasn't there for me… it doesn't seem to be there for him. I manage it (…) uhm (…) well, I'm trying hard to do and I feel like I'm succeeding in making my home for him a place he can trust. But I still see sadness in his life. And (…) it's not the security that I want him to have (…) (…).

T: "I noticed that you used the word sadness about him, and you also used the word sadness about yourself". F: "Maybe he mirrors my feelings with me, and at home with his mum. Because at his mum's he's scared and angry (...) and I spend a lot of time being sad". T: "But if you first say that he is sad and you are sad, and (...) look at his sadness, are there more emotions than sadness in his sadness?" F: "More feelings of sadness in his sadness?" T: "Are there more emotions (...) are there other emotions besides sadness in his sadness?" F: "I don't know if it's that in general or if it's specific. I mean (...). I can remember (...)". T: "When you see that he feels sad, do you think this is pure sadness, or is it mixed with other emotions also in the sadness?" F:

> Mixed emotions! Mixed emotions. I think he's angry sometimes. He's angry and sad at the same time. And sometimes he gets scared. He often starts the two or three days (visit) (...) he often starts with the sad stuff, then they drift towards the anger stuff after a few hours, and it comes out during the first day.

T: "If anger could talk, what would the words be?" F: Oh, lots of things he could say. One would be: "Why did you leave?" Another would be: "You don't act like I'm the most important person in the world to you". T: "I'm sorry". (His ex-wife has stopped typing now and is looking at him intently and listening carefully.) F:

> He will say: "You don't act like I'm the most important person in the world to you". He often asks me questions (...) is basically. (...) well, he tries to feel that he is loved by me (...), it's hard to say the words, but (...). I think I tell him that he is, or: "You are the most important person to me. You are very important to me. There's nobody in the world (...) you know (...) who's more important". All different kinds of ways to say it. Besides the word important. But there's often an answer (...) what mood he's in. Or if he feels a bit closed off (...) he feels (...) it's particularly problematic if I'm going to meet other women. Something that disturbs him deeply. He brings it up quite often.

T: "He doesn't like it?". F:

> He doesn't like it. He doesn't like that he feels he can be left (...) out (...) and maybe I won't see him anymore and won't like him anymore. I could get married and have more children. These are things he comes up with. And speaks. And (...) this is a problem that creates a lot of sadness and some anger. It starts when I pick him up. He always wants to know where I've been and who I've been with the night before and things like that.

T: "Can you tell me?" F: "I'm doing it now". After the meeting, Dad ended his own uncertainty and decided to ask for a formal divorce. She resisted at first, but after the divorce was a fact, she began to figure out her own life and flourished. It's hard to know if there was any connection between these events and the above conversation.

The different steps in a meeting

Exemplified by two meetings between the local therapist, Sara, Anna and Peter (a couple) and one of us.

The local therapist

If it's a consultation with the local therapist and the client, family or network, we first meet with the therapist alone and ask if they would like to talk before the client, family or *network* arrives. It happens, but rarely, that the therapist agrees we should start only when everyone is present. Sara said we could wait until the couple arrived.

The translation

If a translator is needed, the local therapist is asked before the client, family or network arrives whether they prefer to translate. This rarely happens, and they may participate in different editions. When the client, family or network arrives, they are, at the very beginning, asked the same question. Often, they don't understand and are therefore asked: "Do you prefer the translation word for word, or is it better to talk for a while and then do the translation?" Almost always, they prefer the latter. Then to the translator: "Please translate your way!" We don't instruct a specific type of translation.

During the meeting, the client, family or network usually speaks not to us but to the translator, as they soon realise that we neither understand nor receive their words, but the translator does. Therefore, we may occasionally ask the translator: "Did you notice that anything they said was particularly important for them to say?" If the translator has noticed it, we ask him or her to talk more about it. In this way, the translator moves towards the position of therapist.

Sara, Anna, Peter and one of us all spoke English, so no translator was needed.

Do you want to know more about me?

Then we usually ask the client, family or network: "Do you want to know more about me than what you've been told?" We assume that this question can facilitate contact between them and us. One person asked: "What is your therapeutic philosophy?" and, after being told, said with relief: "That is close to our therapists who are in the room". A mum in a family asked: "What are your hobbies?" When they, the family of a daughter currently hospitalised in a mental hospital, were told that their hobby was carpentry, the mother excitedly said that carpentry was also her husband's hobby. Then the father and one of us had a long talk about carpentry. That conversation helped to reduce the strong tension between the father and daughter. Another family asked: "Have you met depressive patients?" and one of us said: "Yes". A family from Colombia asked if they could hear more about Norway. We told them, and we talked about the differences between their country and Norway.

Anna and Peter were probably informed and wanted to talk further.

The history of this meeting

We ask: "Who had the idea for this meeting?" When we find out who it is, we can approach them and ask: "Which of the people here liked your idea of coming here, or was someone reserved?" Talking about this helps us understand who wants to talk and who would rather not. Sara, who had met the couple several times, came up with the idea of asking us to join, and both Anna and Peter appreciated it.

How will you use the meeting?

Sara said she wanted to see the situation from a different perspective and especially to see how one of us participated in the reflective conversation. One of us left the room and went behind the one-way mirror to sit there with the rest of the group. He usually thinks that he has a basket hanging on his arm and puts the words that he sees are important to them in the basket.

The conversation

There was a lot of tension between the two, and their relationship was under threat. When he comes home, he prefers to read the newspaper or watch TV instead of talking to Anna and their two children. He has visited a doctor who diagnosed him with Attention Deficit Hyperactivity Disorder (ADHD), but that didn't stop her from being angry with him.

Peter:

> To what extent has ADHD been a catalyst for that (…) when I was growing (…) when things went wrong because of (…) of brain chemistry (…) I don't know (…) it's almost like a puzzle that… I hope the pill I got will "unlock me" (…) I don't know what it's like to be close (…). I would like to be close (…) this is the only life we have (…).

(He spoke with intensity and had his hands folded behind his neck. If the breathing movements in the abdomen stop, it helps to use your hands in this way to lift the upper part of the chest to get more air. It needs to be noticed – discreetly without commenting). "I can't connect emotionally with my wife and children (…) maybe medicine will help (…) biology is a lot of the reason (…) it has interfered with my emotional development (…)". He is interrupted by Anna: "My anger is an everyday thing (…). I'm angry all the time (…). I feel isolated from Peter (…). I feel like a stranger in my own home (…) he doesn't see me (…)" (To Peter):

> I want to trust you (…). I want you to be my best friend (…). I want to feel more together with you (…) my father was also angry like me (…). I remember as a younger (…) as a young teenager and after that (…). I was always considered a very (…) very (…) very nice girl (…) so nice (…). I was always smiling (…) it

> was so amazing to see me (…) to be around me (…) and I just think (…) which (…) part of it was a game (…) I don't mean all of it (…).

Sara: "Can you tell me more about your father? How did it come that he was an angry person?" Anna:

> He was a very angry man (…) if there was something he didn't like, he could get very angry (…) very angry (…). I remember he bought a big jar and filled it with pickles (…) one day someone broke it (…). I don't know who it did so (…) we ran out (…) my mum ran out and bought another one (…) unfortunately it wasn't the same one.

(She laughs as she speaks and shows with her hands how he threw the jar on the floor). (…) when he came home, and he saw that his jar wasn't there, he took the new jar and threw it on the floor (…). (…) I'll never forget this (Laughs intensely). Sara: "How old were you?" Anna: "Twelve (…)". Peter: "I've seen a lot more anger in my life (…)". Anna: "From your mum?" Peter: "No, I think from my stepfather (…) I laughed when I thought about it (…) from my stepfather and my grandfather". Anna: "They were angry people?" Peter: "(…) I think my grandfather (…)". Anna: "You only lived there for a year?" Peter: Yes, but I don't know the tone of my family (…) what I mean to say (…) is that I have (…) I have pretty good defence mechanisms… I'm never perfect, but (…) so (…) and the condition that I think I told you I have (….) and part of it is that distance (…) and (…) and (…) part of the distance is a protective ability I guess (…) ("Unlock" was repeated three more times with the body in a tense position, and that word went into the "basket").

Bits from the team's reflections

> I heard two big words (…). Anna talked about anger (…) and Peter unlocks (…). I started to ask myself questions about anger (…) is there more emotions in anger than anger (…) and in cases when she is very angry with Peter (…) is there more emotions in anger than anger (…) and I think she (…) when the words spoke out, she started to give answers to my questions (…) because she said I was smiling all the time (…). I was very happy (…) I was a nice child (…) and as she said I had a feeling that there were much more feelings in happiness than just happiness (…) and she pointed to the time her father was very angry (…) had a jar… broke the jar (…) and I thought when she talked like that (…) that maybe her father was so blinded by his anger that he couldn't see how much they had done (…).) to get a new jar (…) he wasn't able to see the efforts of the others to make amends (…) because maybe he had been so blinded by his anger (…)(…) so the word anger came back (…) and I kept asking myself (…) are there more emotions in anger when it comes up between them like anger (…) she talked about fear (…). I wonder if you see more in that word anger when it comes up (…) is there more in there (…) more emotions (…) are the emotions

> coloured (…) what colour (…) is it warm emotions or cold emotions (…) there were questions like that (…).) there was so much in that word (…) is there more to the word than what you see and hear (…)(…) and then the word unlocks from his side (…) it became the big word (…) and I asked myself when it came to dilemmas (…) if you should do the same and if you shouldn't (…).) if you were to do the same thing and look at the word and actually unlock "word unlock" what would you see (…) is it wise to do it at all (…) is the first dilemma (…) should it be unlocked (…) and who should you discuss it with (…) is it wise to unlock it or is it not (…) and if it should be unlocked (…) my thoughts (…) maybe one of the most important is (…) the question: Who should be there to participate (…) to pay attention to him searching into the concern and unlocking if it gets unlocked (…) it's a question of attention: Who should it be (…) who should give him attention (…) if it is wise to unlock it (…) those were my thoughts.

The scene changes The couple and Sara return in front of the mirror

Anna: "I forgot how important this feedback is so (…)(…)" (Long silence as Anna looks away and Peter follows her silently) (…) (whispering "I can't talk (…) it's very (…) it's very emotional (…)(…)". "Sara: (…) you don't have to talk (…)(…) (…)(…)". Anna: (Looking silently to the side for two minutes) (…) (…) it strikes me (…) I see more things after such an interaction (…). Sara: "(…) do you want to share your thoughts?" Anna:

> It was talked about intimacy, and it was talked about unlocking and feeling that this is unlocking (…) it's very interesting to start thinking (…) because we always assume that unlocking is a very positive step forward in our relationship (…) and (…) now I want to release (…) well, it's a step forward for one's own development (…) for example (…). I don't know if it was meant that unlocking was (…) a (…) not a positive thing (…)(…) it can be very negative when it comes to the outcome (…) and (…) I just thought (…) well it's probably very good for oneself, but not good for the others (…) the whole (…).) (…) and then the blindness of anger (…) and the fear in anger (…) it affected me a lot because (…) and then I remember when I went back to Israel I told my father (…) that (…) he doesn't see very well (…) he's 85 (…) and I just told him that he should really see (…) that he should really be happy for me (…).) that he should really be happy that his grandchildren and his children came every day to see him (…) well, he should be one of the happiest people in the world because he has (…) he can't see very well (…) he's 85 and he can't be the guy he wanted to be (…) he should be so happy (…).) he should be so happy (…) he should see how we are so good as a family (…) and that's the blindness (…) I don't know if he just let me see (…) but it's a matter of personality (…) he's always just (…) but the fear (…) the blindness of anger (…) yes (…) and that's true (…).

(Looking at Peter).

> When I'm angry I don't see you (…) I don't see you (…) I don't think that in process I see you (…)(…) even if you did something to annoy me I don't feel that you are harmful (…)(…) if you do something it's because you happen to (…) not know how much it affects me or something like that (…) and (…) I feel that it will continue (…).) I feel it will continue (…)(…) I just keep thinking about anger and blindness (…) that really (…) really helped (…) me very, very (…) it might just be a phase where I understand what my anger is (…) it will be easier for me not to be blind to him (…) so (…) but I really appreciate the group (…).

Anna: "Hey, Peter?". Peter:

> I guess (…) listening to the group I felt on a level privileged (…) so many sensitive, caring people who took the time to look at us and (…) to express their feelings (…) they all communicated a lot of care (…) quite a special experience (…) and (…) it (…) reminded me that I go through most of my life (….) without that feeling element… I felt like I was listening to a discourse in one of the films (…) I watched in my youth (…) it was almost secondary that they were talking about me (…) but there was a sense of connection with mindsets related to how these people feel (…) discourse and (…) feeling (…)(…) a general sense (…). I spend most of my life quite sheltered from that (…) in terms of unlocking and the risk of that I think (…) I don't know (…) influenced by me (…) I'm not sure what she fears (…) was she afraid of wanting to be unlocked?) was she afraid of wanting to be distanced by or I would be distanced by it (…) maybe she would be afraid that I would (…) unlocked would move (…) what influenced you (Talking to Anna) (…) what struck you so powerfully (…) about the comment (…) about the danger of unlocking (…).

Anna:

> That you have to be ready (…) it affected me because (…) it's like a switch (…) you unlock and everything is fine (…) what suddenly struck me, it just opened more doors (…) and it's not necessarily (…) we can expect something (…) that everything will not be so rosy (…) and also be prepared for anything (…).

Peter:

> What do you mean, Anna? Does it mean that (…) it's not necessarily that when you get unlocked that you will be the most happy person in the world (…) or you solve your problem of unlocking (…) you can hit more pain (…) the more I think about it, you will have more pain (…) and you have to be open to (…).

Peter: "I don't know how much of it is ADHD or how much of it is (…) pathology that comes from my own background (…). Peter is familiar with anger, not intimacy (…). I hope the medication will help (…)".

Sara later said that they became more intimate and opened more doors, and Peter longed to be unlocked.

No talking about the client, families or network after the meeting

When the client, families or network leave the meeting, the meeting is over. We strongly discipline ourselves not to talk about the client, families or network after they have left. Sometimes we need to talk about ourselves – what feelings and thoughts are left in us.

Assumptions about reality, living people and language

What I'm writing here is very condensed compared to the sources referred to.

The written sources have been Ludwig Wittgenstein (1953; 1980), von Wright (1990; 1994), Grayling (1988), Gergen (1994), Shotter, 1993a; b; 1996), Lev Vygotsky (1988), Morson (1986), Jacques Derrida (1989), Michael Bakhtin (1990; 1993); Morson (1986); Harold Goolishian (Anderson & Goolishian, 1999).

Collaboration with physiotherapists over the years, especially meetings with Aadel Bülow-Hansen and Gudrun Øvreberg, has had a major influence on the development of these ideas (Øvreberg, 1986; Ianssen, 1997). The sources have also been our own experiences of practising these assumptions. Not least, having participated in a number of reflective processes under very different circumstances has been important in formulating these ideas. Reflective processes are open-ended conversations in which questions and answers come from all the perspectives present (Andersen, 1995).

A few assumptions about reality

Reality consists of three parts: (1) the visible but non-moving, such as a bone in a hand, (2) the visible and moving, such as the hand that in one moment opens and let's go, and in the next moment closes and holds onto something and (3) the invisible but moving, such as the experience of a handshake. We can explain what the leg is, but we can only explain what the hand can be. We don't know what the handshake is, but that's not so important if we feel how we can relate to the person we're shaking hands with. Some would say, "I know what a handshake is; it's a meeting of two hands!" But where does the meeting take place? In the skin? In the touch on the bones? In the look that follows the handshake. Points 1 and 2 can be described so that the mind can understand them. Point 3 can only be experienced by the body. Descriptions of point 1 are best made using numbers, nouns and adjectives, while descriptions of point 2 benefit from verbs. In our attempts to describe point 3, we are most helped by using metaphors that help us feel what we are experiencing.

A few assumptions about people

The first thing we do in life is to breathe in, with holy words; breathe in, before the first scream comes. The last thing we do in life is to give (spirit) out; let the spirit go. Between the first breath in and the last breath out, the breath goes continuously; inhalation after exhalation after inspiration after exhalation and so on. When something happens to us, the inhalation movements are affected: "I lost my breath", "I gasped", "I got a lump in my throat", "My stomach hurts" (when the breathing movements in the stomach stop) etc.

The exhaling movements help many of the expressions, such as the emotions and words that are reactions to what we feel. They can be talking, laughing, crying, shouting and so on. The baby's first cry is a response to facing the cold reality outside. It was warmer and more comfortable in the mother's womb. Those around the child hear the cry and give back what the child needs to stop crying. Bakhtin thought that life was a constant responding activity. One person's expression is a response to another's just-given expression. He said, "The soul is a gift that my spirit gives to the other" (Bakhtin, 1990, p. 132). The soul is the meeting place where one's expression (spirit) is received by the other and responded to by the other's expression (spirit). One's contribution to the soul, which lies between the one and the other person, is to receive and respond to the other's expression. Receiving and responding are sacred and serious activities.

Ten assumptions about language

1 Language is defined here as all expressions that are of great importance in the common perspective between people. They are of many kinds, such as speaking, writing, painting, dancing, singing, pointing, crying, laughing, screaming, hitting, etc. When these expressions, which are bodily, take place in the presence of others, language becomes a social activity. Our expressions are social offers to be able to participate in community with others.
2 We need the expressions to create meanings. If one of the expressions, such as words or speaking, is not available, another type of expression, such as painting, can make it possible to create meaning.
3 The expressions come first, and then the meaning follows. This is created. Harry Goolishian used to say, "We don't know what we're thinking until we've said it".
4 The meaning is in the expression, not underneath or behind it. The meanings in the expressions, such as in the words, are very personal. Some of the words, when we hear them, will bring us back to and make us relive something we have experienced before.
5 The expressions are informative, which means they tell something about us to others and to ourselves. Now, I believe that when I speak out loud, I am primarily speaking to myself. Since the words I express are so strongly linked to my understanding, by listening carefully to what I say, I can examine my own

understanding. Expressions are also formative. We become who we become when we express ourselves the way we do. It would be more appropriate to say, "Grandad always did something kind, so he was kind all the time", rather than saying "Grandad was kind" or "Grandad had so much kindness". By using verbs to be and by not including time and context, it's easy to become mesmerised by your own statement and believe that what you're describing is static: "Grandpa is kind, he has that character", or "Grandpa has a lot of kindness, he has a kind personality". When we talk to ourselves like this, we can easily get the idea that a person has both character and personality.

6 The expressions, both in inner and personal conversations and in outer and social conversations, are accompanied by movements. Those that follow inner conversations are smaller and nuanced, while those that follow outer conversations are larger, such as waving hands. Sometimes both therapists and researchers misunderstand when they say that the spoken word does not match the body language; for example, when someone says, "I'm so happy", with a sad expression. As I see it, the words "I'm so happy" are the social offer to bond with the other person, while the sad face belongs to an inner and probably sad conversation that the person is probably not interested in sharing with the other person. Therefore, if the other person does not want to share their inner conversation, I see it as common courtesy neither to see how the inner conversation is presented in their body expressions. It should be an ongoing task for the therapist and researcher to evaluate which of a person's expressions are offers to participate in social bonds and which are not. Laurence Singh, a psychotherapist I met, offered me a phrase, "A social offer". It's used to describe expressions that contribute to a social bond, as opposed to expressions that are personal and not meant for a social bond.

7 The movements of the expressions, not least the breathing movements that form and produce the inner and outer voices, are personal. Breathing movements are as personal as fingerprints. Lev Vygotsky said, "We are the voices that have inhabited us" (Morson, 1986, p. 8). Perhaps one can nuance it to: "We are the movements that form and produce the voices that have inhabited us".

8 In his time, Heraclitus said, "Everything is changing, but the change takes place according to an immutable law (logos), and this law involves a mutual interaction between opposites, but still so that the interaction between the various forces produces a harmony in total" (Skirbekk, 1980, p. 29). Perhaps you can dare to make some small changes, like: "A person is moving, but the movements are happening..." Or even: "A person is movement, but..." When we stand, and stand in balance, the muscles that bend at the knees and hips are active at the same time as the muscles that extend the knees and hips are active.

9 When you speak out loud, you say something to both others and yourself. Now, I think the most important person I'm talking to is myself. As mentioned in point 5, expressions are formative and shape our understanding. Ludwig Wittgenstein and Georg Henrik von Wright wrote that our own speech enchants

our understanding. We cannot be mesmerised by our own speech. When we belong to a society, such as a professional society, we absolutely must speak the language of that society. You must be willing to be occupied by that language if you want to stay there. If this language uses the verbs to be and to have without indicating context and time at the same time, then, as said earlier, one can easily understand that people are static. Different types of language, such as the language of competition, the language of strategic management, the language of pathology, etc., all have their consequences, both for those who are described and for those who describe.

10 In 1985, Harry (Harold) Goolishian launched the concept of "The problem-created system". He said that a problematic situation quickly attracts the attention of many people.

The attracted people usually pose the questions: "How can I understand this?" and "What should I do?" Maria doesn't want to go to school anymore. It is an example of a problem that creates opinions in others; a system of opinions is created. If two or more people have the same opinion, a conversation will easily make them repeat and confirm the opinion, and very little that is new is developed. If two or more people have somewhat different opinions and can listen to each other, a conversation between them will easily create new and useful opinions. If two or more people have very different opinions, they may find it difficult to listen to each other and may even interrupt and correct each other. When that doesn't happen often, the conversations merge, and if it does happen often, a big problem is created.

Language is all kinds of expression – also expressive movement without words, even without sounds

Creating a counselling exercise that increases the therapist's relational sensitivities

We are of the opinion that dealing with others, for example in therapy, is to be in the moving and invisible part of reality. This part consists of encounters, and as Bakhtin said, every encounter is "a once-occurring being-event". We cannot, therefore, fully generalise from one encounter to another, but we can learn from one encounter what not to do in a later encounter. The following co-research aims to achieve that ambition.

Two summaries: (1) It seems that the better the relationship between clients and therapists, the better the outcome for the clients, which means a change to a better life. The technique or theory that the therapist brings is of less importance (Lambert et al., 1986; Lambert, 1989; Duncan et al., 1994). (2) By far, the majority of psychotherapists argue that their ongoing collaboration with clients and their discussions of their practical work with colleagues are the most useful sources for their development as a therapist. A fairly small proportion said that research articles or presentations on psychotherapy were the most important sources (Morrow-Bradley et al., 1986; Cohen et al., 1986; Hosmand et al., 1992).

Together with two teams, one in Northern Norway and one in Stockholm, we collaborated to develop a useful research practice. This is described in Andersen (1995b; 1997), and the corresponding thoughts on such research practice in Andersen (1996a; 1998) are discussed. If our research process were to be linked to an earlier research tradition, it would be Participatory Action Research (Whyte, 1991).

The initial idea was that the therapists would meet all the clients sometime after the treatment had ended and, through conversation, find out what it had been like for the clients to be in therapy.

We soon realised that not all clients were ready for such a conversation. Some said that they had finally managed to put the period of problems behind them. They saw such a conversation as a risk of bringing back the troubled feelings from that problematic period. A few said that they disliked their relationship with the therapists so much that they did not want to meet them again. Some found it too cumbersome for practical reasons to return. Quite a few came. We developed the safest possible procedure. Firstly, when therapy ends, the therapists will tell the clients that they (the therapists) will call them after a certain period to see how they are doing. When the therapist calls, it will be safest to begin the telphonic conversation by asking if it is okay to have a short conversation about how their life situation is now and to talk about what it was like afterwards to have participated in therapeutic meetings. In cases where clients felt that the meetings were difficult or uncomfortable, therapists will ask if they would like to come back to talk about it. The therapist explains that such a review can help them learn what is not useful in therapy. Similarly, in cases where therapists themselves have defined therapeutic encounters as difficult or uncomfortable, they will invite clients to come and talk about those encounters.

Conversations about therapeutic conversations

The conversations, which take place sometime (for example, 6 or 12 or 24 months) after the treatment collaboration has ended, consist of three actors: the clients, the therapist and a visiting colleague (an "outsider").

The therapists start the meeting by making it clear that the idea for the meeting came from them (the therapists): "The idea for us (the clients and the therapists) to come together is to clarify what of the therapeutic encounters contributed to the better and what to the worse for you (the clients)". The "outsider" has then referred to research literature that points out that the relationship and cooperation between clients and therapists is important. Then he or she might say:

> To allow as much space as possible for the nuances of your collaboration, I suggest that I first talk to you as a therapist, since you had the idea for this meeting. Then I'll talk to you, the clients, about the thoughts you get when you listen to

> my conversation with the therapists. Then I'll talk to the therapist about their response to our conversation. We will all always be together in this room. You will alternate between being part of the talking and listening to what the others are saying.

Some may find that this approach is a variant of reflective processes (Andersen, 1991, 1992).

Talk about the process and not the content

Sometimes clients want to talk about issues they once worked on in therapy. In that case, the visiting colleague can instead suggest that they bring this up with their therapist and continue talking about the issues with them. The colleague should avoid becoming a therapist, as this is not what they have been asked to help with. It is important for the colleague to remember that the questions and comments made are not only heard by the person they are speaking to, but also by others who are present.

In a therapeutic process, with clients and therapists present, the focus is on how clients can be in the world in different ways. In this counselling process, with clients, therapists and the outsider, the focus is on how therapists can be-in-the-world-as-therapists in different ways. The conversation itself is no different from that of therapy. It must be assumed that some answers to the various questions may create unease and cause the listeners to have unpleasant experiences. In such cases, the colleague must proceed very slowly and keep all senses focused on all parties to notice the small signs that indicate what is too difficult to talk about and/or hear. These small signs are the ones we all recognise: a movement of the chair, a furrowed brow, a look in the eyes, a cough, etc. If such signs appear, the outsider can break the questions down into even smaller and more detailed ones. He should remember that questions of this kind should sometimes only be raised and eventually thought about, not necessarily answered.

The visiting colleague first speaks to the therapist, while the clients listen to the conversation. Here are a few examples of general opening questions for the therapists (and remember that the questions also reach the clients' ears):

> What did you have in mind when you asked the clients to come today? What of your contributions to the therapy sessions do you think the clients appreciated most? If you had to find some words to describe the work you did together, what would they be? Were there times when the meetings were too unusual for them? Could there be something they would have liked to talk about but never discussed? Were there moments you remember that were difficult for yourself? Were there times when you yourself had thoughts that you never revealed, but in retrospect thought it would have been useful to talk about? Was this therapy like the therapies you've had with other clients, or was it different?

These questions give the therapist the opportunity to open up about their own thoughts or feelings that may have arisen during the therapy. These were never thematised then or after the therapy ended. There may be struggles in the therapeutic relationship, or the therapists may be lecturing, strategic or manipulative, or they may be too involved or too intimate. They may also be attracted to one of the clients and not others, or the therapy may be impacting the therapist's life outside the therapy room. It can be extremely difficult for therapists to find answers that they and their clients are able to hear. The "outsider" must therefore allow the therapists to take all the time they need to find different answers.

If the therapists find answers, the colleague can continue with questions like:

> If, in the therapeutic sessions you once had together, you were to talk to the clients... about this or that..., how could you have done it? If the clients were ready to talk about it, how do you think they would have wanted to talk about it?

This is followed by a conversation between the clients and the "outsider" with the therapist listening. Here are some examples of questions that can be discussed with the clients:

> Would you like to comment on what you heard during the conversation between the therapists and me? We talked about (this or that), what are your thoughts on that? In addition to what the therapists want to talk about, is there anything you want to talk about? Is there anything special you remember from the therapeutic meetings? Were there times when the meetings were of little interest to you? Were there times when you wanted to talk about something you never got to talk about? Were there times when you tried to say something they didn't hear?

The therapists then comment on what they have just heard.

Three examples

A male therapist asked a female client to come in for a "catch-up" session two years after they last met. She had stopped therapy after two meetings without telling the therapist why. When the "outsider" asked the therapist what it was that the client wanted the therapy to be like, he couldn't remember. The client could. She said that after years of doubt, she finally decided to consult a female family doctor to talk about her difficulties. She felt that the doctor fulfilled her (the client's) wishes, but the doctor felt that she was not good enough and referred the client to the psychiatric clinic. The client hesitantly accepted when the doctor emphasised in his written referral that the client needed to see a female therapist. That didn't happen, and she left after two meetings with the male therapist. In a painful period after this happened, she began to write, at first, incoherent notes that indicated chaos, fear and little hope. However, the notes became more and more coherent, and writing to herself helped her find a new balance. The male therapist, listening intently to the story, never again forgot to ask his clients, "What is the story behind the idea of coming to therapy?" The client's telling of her story, with the therapist as a witness, made the woman leave the "after-talk" with a feeling of having regained her dignity.

A team of three reunites with a family of three (mum, dad and son) and a visiting "outsider" one year after treatment. The therapists said that the conversations were often such that the son did not attend. The therapists were asked if they had ever considered the possibility of meeting the son without his parents. "No", they said, "it was impossible". However, the boy told them that coming alone was what he wanted. The therapists were shocked by their own rigour in answering: "No, it was impossible". The feeling of being strict remained with them long after that meeting. Although the team was always open to change, they said the conversation had introduced much more flexibility into their work. Not only did they start discussing with families how to work together, but the team itself began to vary the format. Sometimes all three worked together, sometimes just two, alternating between two and one depending on the families they met.

A team consisting of one female and one male therapist met with a couple and the "outsider" one year after the treatment ended. The therapists wondered what it was like for the man in the couple, who was very talkative, to be stopped in the meeting by the male therapist. The therapist said that he had to do that in order to make room for the man's wife. If she hadn't been heard, they were afraid she would leave the marriage. The husband said that it was difficult for him to be interrupted. Often, he left the meetings with a lump in his throat. The visiting colleague asked the man what the words would be if his throat could speak in such cases. "Help me", he said, almost crying. The male therapist later said that this was an example of what an "outsider" should not do, namely, to work therapeutically. In addition, it made it possible for the man to experience it as better therapy than what the male therapist himself had been able to provide. The male therapist said to the visiting colleague: "What you could have asked the man, and what I would have accepted, was: "What could your male therapist have done so that your unexpressed feelings could come out into the open?"

We learnt that the outsider must ask open questions and avoid expressing opinions about the previous therapeutic collaboration. The visiting colleague must be concerned with *the how*, understood as how the clients and therapists worked together. Focusing on what they talked about in therapy should only be done to shed light on how they had worked together. For therapists to talk like this about their work with clients, with them present, and they themselves then talk about the clients' experiences, is both extremely demanding and extremely rewarding. The high intensity of the meeting was particularly mentioned. The therapist said that their own listening to their own answers, with the clients as witnesses, had a great impact on them (the therapists). The knowledge developed in such processes is emotionally charged knowledge that moves the therapist to a different position as a therapist; towards more sensitivity to their own experiences and to their experiences of being with clients. This knowledge is first felt in the body before it reaches the rational understanding of that which gives meaning, and before it becomes part of the therapist's repertoire in practice.

This process of re-searching together with clients is so energy-intensive that it can't happen too often. On the other hand, its impact is so profound that the two teams who helped develop this process said that two such meetings a year were sufficient. The procedure will hopefully stimulate the therapist's sensitivity to understanding what clients want to talk about and how they want to talk about it. If the therapist thereby becomes the one who follows the clients and only engages in what the clients want the therapist to be engaged in, it will most likely be easier for the therapist to recognise their own thoughts and feelings. Conflicts and tensions will diminish, and the therapist will become less wilful and less easily caught up in their own feelings and experiences of the situation, the clients and themselves.

References

Aaltonen, J., Seikkula, J. & Lehtinen, K. (1997). *Comprehensive Open Dialogue Approach and the Incidence of Schizophrenia and Prodromal Patients: The Western Lapland Project*. Unpublished manuscript.

Andersen, T. (1987). The reflecting team: Dialogue and meta-dialogue in clinical work. *Family Process, 26*(4), 415–428.

Andersen, T. (1988). Change knows its own way. In H. Hårtveit, A. Johnsen & S. Tømmerås (Eds.), *Through the Looking Glass and Back: Reflections on Systems in Treatment, Treatment Systems and Systemic Treatment*. Oslo: Tano.

Andersen, T. (1991). *The Reflecting Team*. New York: W.W. Norton.

Andersen, T. (1992a). Relationship, language and pre-understanding in the reflecting process. *Australian and New Zealand Journal of Family Therapy, 13*(2), 87–91.

Andersen, T. (1992b). Inter-human relationships, language and pre-understanding. *Focus on the Family, 92*(1), 33–43.

Andersen, T. (1995a). Reflecting processes; Acts of informing and forming: You can borrow my eyes, but you must not take them away from me! In S. Friedman (Ed.), *The Reflective Process in Action*. New York: The Guilford Press.

Andersen, T. (1995b). Clients and therapists as co-researchers to increase therapist sensitivity. *Focus on the Family, 4*, 193–200.

Andersen, T. (1996a). Research of treatment practice; What should or what ought to or what can such a practice be? *Focus on the Family, 1*, 3–16.

Andersen, T. (1996b). Language is not innocent. In F. Kaslow (Ed.), *Handbook of Relational Diagnosis* (pp. 119–125). New York, Chichester, Brisbane, Toronto, Singapore: John Wiley & Sons.

Andersen, T. (2001). The significance of expressions in treatment and research; some preliminary formulations. In E. Kjellberg (Ed.), *Man kan inte så noga väta ... Barnpsykiatriska utredningar tilsamans med socialtjänsten. Practice and research through open dialogue and reflective processes*. Stockholm: Mareld.

Anderson, H. & Goolishian, H. (1988). A view of human systems as linguistic systems: Some preliminary and evolving ideas about the implications for clinical theory. *Family Process, 27*, 371–393.

Anderson, H. & Goolishian, H. (1992). *Från påverkan til medverkan*. Stockholm: Mareld.

Anderson, H. & Jensen, P. (2008). *Inspirations. Tom Andersen and reflective processes*. Oslo: Gyldendal Akademisk.

Bakhtin, M. (1990). *Art and Answerability: Early Philosophical Essays*. Austin: University of Texas Press.

Bakhtin, M. (1993). *Toward a Philosophy of the Act*. Austin: University of Texas Press.

Bateson, G. (1978). The birth of a matrix or double bind and epistemology. In M. M. Berger (Ed.), *Beyond the Double Bind*. New York: Brunner/Mazel.

Bateson, G. (1979). *Steps to an Ecology of Mind*. Chicago: University of Chicago Press.

Cohen, L. H., Sargent, M. M. & Sechrest, L. B. (1986). Use of psychotherapy research by professional psychologists. *American Psychologist, 41*(2), 198–206.

D'Andrade, R. (1986). Three scientific world views and the covering law model. In D. W. Fiske & E. Schweder (Eds.), *Metatheory in Social Science*. Chicago: The University of Chicago Press.

Danielsen, E. (1997). *Vygotsky. The Mozart of psychology*. Copenhagen: Danish Psychological Publishers.

Duncan, B., Hubble, M. & Rusk, G. (1994). To intervene or not to intervene? That is not the Question. *Journal of Systemic Therapy, 13*(4), 22–30.

Edwardsson, M. (1994). Open sesame! Utredningsarbeid innom barnpsykiatrisk öppenvård. *Focus on the Family, 3*, 181–191.

Finne, I. (1997). *The child's psychiatric disorder or Olav's difficult life?* Bodø: Unpublished manuscript.

Forsberg, G. & Wallmark, J. (1998). *Nätverksboken - om mötets mögighet*. Stockholm, Sweden: Liber.

Gergen, K. (1985). The social constructionist movement in modern psychology. *American Psychologist, 40*, 266–275.

Gergen, K. (1990). Therapeutic professions and the diffusions of deficit. *Journal of Mind and Behaviour, 11*(3), 353–386.

Gergen, K. (1994a). *Realities and Relationships*. London: Sage Harvard University Press.

Gergen, K. (1994b). *Toward Transformation in Social Knowledge* (2nd ed.). London: Sage.

Grayling, A. C. (1988). *Wittgenstein*. New York: Oxford University Press.

Groth, Ö. (1994). *Nordkalotten, Konung Faravids Land*. Stockholm: Tidens förlag.

Haarakangas, K. (1997). The voices in treatment meeting. A dialogical analysis of the treatment meeting conversations in family-centered psychiatric treatment process in regard to the team activity. English Summary. Diss. *Jyväskylä Studies in Education, psychology and Social Research, 130*, 119–126.

Hansen, V. (1987). Psychiatric service within primary care. *Acta Psychiatrica Scandinavica, 76*, 121–128.

Hoshmand, L. T. & Polkinghorne, D. (1992). Redefining the science-practice relationship and professional training. *American Psychologist, 47*(1), 55–66.

Ianssen, B., Øvreberg, G., Andersen, T., Hanssen, I., Kvebæk, I., Ottesen, A. & Rongved, E. (1997). *Movement, Life and Change. In the Footsteps of Aadel Bülow-Hansen*. Oslo: Cappelen Akademisk Forlag.

Jensen, P. (2008). Crossroads. In H. Anderson & P. Jensen (Eds.), *Inspirations. Tom Andersen and reflective processes* (pp. 192–209). Oslo: Gyldendal Akademisk.

Johnson, M. (1987). *The Body in the Mind*. Chicago: Chicago University Press.

Karlsson, B. & Borg, M. (2017). *Recovery. Traditions, Renewals and Practices*. Oslo: Gyldendal Akademisk.

Keränen, J. (1992). The choice between outpatient and inpatient treatment in a family centred psychiatric treatment system. English Summary. Diss. *Jyväskylä Studies in Education, Psychology and Social Research, 93*, 124–129.

Kjellberg, E. (1995). Using the reflecting process with families stuck in violence and child abuse. In S. Friedman (Ed.), *The Reflecting Team in Action* (pp. 38–61). New York: The Guilford Press.

Kjellberg, E. (1999). *Man kan inte så noga väta ... Barnpsykiatriska utredningar tilsamans med socialtjänsten. Practice and research through open dialogue and reflective processes*. Stockholm: Mareld.
Kolberg, C. (1998). *Basic Features of Paul Ricoeur's hermeneutics with Emphasis on the Ideas of Concrete Reflection and Detour* (Undergraduate thesis in philosophy). Unpublished thesis. University of Tromsø.
Kolstad, A. (ed.) (1995). *On the Trail of the Infinite. A Debate Book on Emmanuel Levinas*. Oslo: H. Aschehougs forlag.
Kvale, S. (1997). *The Qualitative Research Interview*. Oslo: ad Notam.
Lambert, M. J. (1989). The individual therapist's contribution to psychotherapy process and outcome. *Clinical Psychology Review, 9*, 469–485.
Lambert, M. J., Shapiro, D. A. & Bergin, A. E. (1986). The effectivesness of psychotherapy. In S. Garfield & A. Bergin (Eds.), *Handbook of Psychotherapy and Behaviour Change*. New York: Wiley.
Lindseth, A. (1988). Pedagogical science? In R. Fjelland, A. Lindseth, I. M. Nilsen & A. Måseide (Eds.), *Treng vi faget pedagogikk?* Oslo: Solum forlag.
Lindseth, A. (1998). *Process and product*. Lecture at the June seminar 15–17 June 1998 at Dundret, Gällivare under the auspices of "Development Project in Systemic Work in the Northern Calotte".
Lundholm, K. O., Östen, J., Groth, R. & Petterson, Y. (1996). *North Scandinavian History*. Stockholm: Tidens förlag.
Lysack, M. (2004). *Reflecting Processes as Practitioner Education in Andersen and White through the Lenses of Bakhtin and Vygotsky* (Unpublished doctoral thesis).Montreal: McGill University.
Maturana, H. (1978). The biology of language: The epistemology of reality. In G. Millerand & E. Lennenberg (Eds.), *Psychology and Biology of Language and Thought*. New York: A.P.
Morgan, G. (1983). Exploring choice. In G. Morgan (Ed.), *Beyond Method*. London: Newbury Park.
Morrow-Beadley, C. & Elliott, R. (1986). Utilization of psychotherapy research by practicing psychotherapists. *American Psychologist, 41*(2), 188–197.
Morson, A. C. (1986). *Bakhtin. Essays and Dialogues on His Work*. Chicago and London: The University of Chicago Press.
Måseide, A. (ed) (1988). *Treng vi faget pedagogikk?* Oslo: Solum forlag.
Oddli, H. W. & Kjøs, P. (1998). *Psychology and science. Modern and postmodern understanding of therapy*. Oslo: Tano Aschehoug.
Penn, P. & Frankfurt, M. (1994). Creating a participant text: Writing, multiple voices, narrative multiplicity. *Family Process, 33*(3), 217–232.
Polkinghorne, D. (1983). *Methodology for the Human Sciences. Systems of Inquiry*. New York: State University of New York Press.
Polkinghorne, D. (1988). *Narrative Knowing and the Human Sciences*. Albany: State University of New York Press.
Reichelt, E. (1996). The duck shear bar. In *Festskrift til professor Tom Andersen på hans 60-årsdag*. ISM's publication series, no. 35. University of Tromsø.
Reichelt, S. (1996). Research for practice - of academic relevance? *Journal of the Norwegian Psychological Association, 33*, 1134–1142.
Sampson, E. E. (1989). The deconstruction of the self. In J. Shotter & K. Gergen (Eds.), *Texts of Identity*. London: Sage Publication.
Seikkula, J. (1991). Family-hospital boundary system in the social network. English summary. Diss. *Jyväskylä Studies in Education, Psychology and Social Research, 80*, 227–232.

Seikkula, J. (1993). The aim of therapy is generating dialogue: Bakhtin and in family session. *Human Systems, 4*, 33–48.
Seikkula, J. (1994). When the boundary opens: Family and hospital in co-evolution. *Journal of Family Therapy, 16*, 401–414.
Seikkula, J. (1995a). From monologue to dialogue in consultation with larger systems. *Human Systems, 6*, 21–42.
Seikkula, J. (1995b). Treating psychosis by means of open dialogue. In S. Friedman (Ed.), *The Reflecting Team in Action*. New York/London: The Guilford Press.
Seikkula, J. (1996). *Open dialogue. From monologue to living dialogue in the social network*. Stockholm: Mareld.
Seikkula, J. (1999). *Open Conversations. Textbook in network therapy*. Oslo: Tano-Aschehoug.
Seikkula, J., Aaltonen, J. & Alakare, B. (1996). Treating psychosis in Western Lapland: Reflective processes and open dialogue instead of hospitalisation and heavy medication. In *Reflection and Dialogue. Festschrift on Tom Andersen's 60th birthday*. ISM Skriftserie, no 35.
Seikkula, J., Aaltonen, J., Alakare, B., Haarakangas, K., Keränen, J. & Sutela, M. (1995). Treating psychosis by means of open dialogue. In S. Friedman (Ed.), *The Reflecting Team in Action*. New York: The Guilford Press.
Seikkula, J., Aaltonen, J., Alakare, B., Holma, J., Lehtinen, V. & Rasinkangas, A. (1997). *Home Treatment by Open Dialogue in First Episode Psychosis: A Two Year Follow-Up on Avoiding Hospitalisation and Neuroleptic Medication*. Western Lapland Project. Unpublished manuscript.
Seikkula, J. & Arnkil, T. (2013). *Open Dialogue in Relational Practice. Respect for Otherness in the Moment*. Oslo: Gyldendal Akademisk.
Seikkula, J. & Sutela, M. (1990). Coevolution of the family and the hospital: The System of boundary. *Journal of Strategic and Systemic Therapies, 9*, 34–42.
Selvini Palazolli, M., Cecchin, G., Boscolo, L. & Prata, G. (1980). Hypothecation-circularity-neutrality: Three guidelines for the conductor of the session. *Family Process, 19*, 3–12.
Shotter, J. (1993a). *Cultural Politics of Everyday Life*. Buckingham: Open University Press.
Shotter, J. (1993b). *Conversational Realities*. London, New York: Sage Publishing.
Shotter, J. (1996). *Some useful quotations from Wittgenstein, Vygotsky, Bakhtin and Volosinov*. Presented at the Sulitjelma conference in North Norway, June 13–15 1996.
Shotter, J. (2004). *On the Edge of Social Constructionism: 'Withness'-Thinking versus Aboutness-Thinking*. Available for purchase by contacting info@kccfoundation.com
Shotter, J. (2005). *Wittgenstein in Practice: His Philosophy of Beginnings, and Beginnings, and Beginnings*. Available for purchase by contacting info@kccfoundation.com
Skirbekk, G. (1980). *History of Philosophy I*. Oslo: Universitetsforlaget.
University of Tromsø (1993). *Festschrift to Professor Tom Andersen on his 60th birthday*. ISM's publication series, no. 35. University of Tromsø.
von Wright, G. H. (1990). Wittgenstein and the twentieth century. In L. Haaparanta (Ed.), *Language, Knowledge and Intentionality*. Helsinki: Acta Philosophica Fennica 49.
von Wright, G. H. (1991). *Science and Reason*. Oslo: Cappelens Akademiske forlag.
von Wright, G. H. (1994). *The Myth of Progress*. Stockholm: Bonnier.
Vygotsky, L. (1988). *Thought and Language*. Cambridge, MA: MIT Press.
Wachthauser, B. R. (1986). History and language in understanding. In B. R. Wachthauser (Ed.), *Hermeneutics and Modern Philosophy*. Albany: State University of New York Press.

Wagner, J. (1998a). Conversations within the walls. Retrospectives and reflections. *Focus on the Family, 3*, 131–144.

Wagner, J. (1998b). Are dialogical conversations possible behind WALLS? Reflections and review. *Human Systems, 9*(2), 95–113.

Wagner, J. & Andersson, T. (1997). *What does the region want to know about the dialogue activities at KVA in Kalmar* (Stensil). Kalmar: Kriminalvårdsmyndigheten i Kalmar.

Warncke, G. (1987). *Gadamer: Hermeneutics, Tradition and Reason*. Stanford, CA: Stanford University Press.

Watzlawick, P., Jackson, D. & Beavin, J. (1967). *Pragmatics of Human Communication. A Study of Interactional Patterns, Pathologies and Paradoxes*. New York: Norton.

Whyte, W. F. (1991). *Participatory Action Research*. London: Sage.

Wittgenstein, L. (1953). *Philosophical Investigations*. Oxford: Blackwell.

Wittgenstein, L. (1980). *Culture and Value*. Oxford: Blackwell.

Øvreberg, G. (ed.) (1986). *Aadel Bülow-Hansen's Physiotherapy*. Tromsø, Oslo: In commission with Norli forlag.

John Shotter on Tom Andersen:

A. Shotter, J. (2007). Not to forget Tom Andersen's way of being Tom Andersen: The importance of what "just happens" to us. *Human Systems: The Journal of Systemic Consultation & Management, 18*(2007), 15–28.

B. Shotter, J. (2010). Movements of feeling and moments of judgement: Towards an ontological social constructionism. *International Journal of Action Research, 6*(1), 16–42. https://nbn-reolving.org/urn:nbn:de0168-ssoar-385068

C. Shotter, J. (2012). Bodily way-finding our way into the future: Finding the guidance we need for our next step within the taking our present step. *Journal of Mental Health Work, 9*(2), 133–143.

D. Shotter, J. (2015). Tom Andersen, fleeting events, the bodily feelings tehy arose in us, and the dialogical: Transitory understnadings and action guiding anticipations. *Australian & New Zealand Journal of Family Theraphy, 36*, 72–87. Doi: 10.1002/anzf.1087

E. Vedeler, A. H. (2007). The worried irrigation man. John Shotter on Tom Andersen in conversation with Anne Hedvig Vedeler. *Focus on the Family, 35*(3), 166–178.

Appendices

Tom Andersen's bibliography collected and edited by Petter H. Næsje

In 1997, Tom Andersen gave me a list of what he had written. I started collecting what I came across of what he had written up until then. This interest has continued to this day. After Tom's death on 15 May 2007, I wanted to make an overview of what I have found that has been published in Norwegian, Swedish, Danish and English. The book *The Reflecting Team: Dialogues and Dialogues about the Various Dialogues* (1990) has been published in at least 11 different languages. Just not in Norwegian.

This bibliography is intended to help those who want to delve deeper into what Tom Andersen has written and said in interviews. In an article in Utposten 1991, Tom introduces himself by saying: About myself: "Former district doctor, now psychiatrist. Restless and doubtful and constantly searching". The bibliography was compiled by Petter H. Næsje with the help of his colleague Morten Hammer and the always interested and helpful specialist library at the Regional Centre for Child and Adolescent Mental Health – South and East.

As an aid to the reader, several articles were published in several different editions, with only minor changes. Several have been published in many different languages. Petter Næsje received some manuscripts from Tom Andersen long before they were published. Articles and books marked with * have co-authors.

1975

Tom Andersen (1975). Physical and mental illness in a Lapp and Norwegian population. Social, somatic and psychiatric studies of geographically defined populations. *Acta Psychiatrica Scandinavica Supplementum, 263*(63), 47–53.

1978

Tom Andersen (1978). Ill Health in two contrasting societies, particularly non-psychiatric morbidity among those with a psychiatric diagnosis. *Psychotherapy and Psychosomatics, 32*, 249–256.

1984

Tom Andersen (1984). The cybernetic way of understanding and its significance for work with mental problems. *Focus on the Family, 1*(1984), 21–31.

Tom Andersen (1984). Consultation: Would you like co-evolution instead of referral? *Family systems medicine, Winter 1984, 2*(4), 370–379.

1985

Tom Andersen (1985). Circular questioning and shifting relationships. An attempt to describe the process of change in family and evaluate the therapy's influence on the changes*. *The Australian, New Zealand Journal of Family Therapy, 6*(3), 145–150.

1986

Tom Andersen (1986). Practice sketches and feedback loops. Four hearts and four families in dilemma*. *Family Systems Medicine, Spring 1986, 4*(1).

Tom Andersen (1986). *Anne and Johanne. A story that provides an opportunity to discuss how life events and life performances can be understood in at least two ways*. Lecture at the Norwegian Women's Health Association's national meeting in Alta on 27 June 1986.

Tom Andersen (1986). Two relatively chaotic situations. *Focus on the Family, 14*, 143–151.

1987

Tom Andersen (1987). Questions created new questions at Skogsholmen in Vega. Harlene Anderson and Harry Goolishian of the Galveston Family Institute, Texas, conducted a seminar for counsellors and future counsellors 23–28 June 1987. *Focus on the Family, 4*(1987), 209–216.

Tom Andersen (1987). The reflecting team: Dialogue and meta-dialogue in clinical work. *Family Process, 26*(4), 415–428.

Tom Andersen (1987). *The reflecting team. A conversation is followed by a conversation about the conversation which is followed by a conversation about the conversation about the conversation.* First Nordic Congress on Family Therapy, Lindkjöping 13–15 August. 1987.

Tom Andersen (1987). The general practitioner and consulting psychiatrist as a team with "stuck" families. *Family Systems Medicine, Winter 1987, 5*(4), 468–481.

1988

Tom Andersen (1988). How can clinical work with systems, e.g. families, be described and understood? Preparations for a Greek kitchen in the Arctic. *Focus on the Family, 1*(1988), 3–5.

Tom Andersen (1988). Change knows its own time and its own ways. In H. Hårtveit, A. Johnsen & S. Tømmerås (eds.). *Through the looking glass and back*. Oslo: Tano.

Tom Andersen (1988). A community-orientated psychiatric health service in Massachusetts, USA. *Nordic Psychiatric Journal, 42*, 225–228.

1989

Tom Andersen (1989). Back and forth and beyond. *The Australian, New Zealand Journal of Family Therapy, 10*, 75–76.

1990

Tom Andersen (1990). *The reflecting team: dialogues and dialogues about the various dialogues*. New York, London: W.W. Norton.

1991

Tom Andersen (1991). *The reflecting team: dialogues and dialogues about the dialogues*. Kent UK: Borgman Publ.

Tom Andersen (1991). Relationships, language and pre-understanding. Some main points from a workshop at Vettre 2 February 1991. *Metaforum*, 19–31.

Tom Andersen (1991). The expressed words create the person. *Utposten, 20*, 196–198.

Tom Andersen (1991). *Social justice and mental health*. Paper read at 3rd World Family Therapy Congress, Finland 2–6 June (Comment: Only an abstract from before the lecture is available here).

Tom Andersen (1991). *The reflective team. Conversations and conversations about conversations*. Stockholm, Sweden: Mareld.

1992

Tom Andersen (1992). From influence to participation. Foreword in H. Anderson & H. Goolishian, *Från påverkan til medverkan*. Stockholm: Mareld. (Comment: From operation to co-operation English edition of the same foreword written at the same time as the one above. Received privately).

Tom Andersen (1992). Reflections on reflecting with families. In S. McNamee & K. Gergen (eds.), *Therapy as Social Construction*. London: Sage publications.

Tom Andersen (1992). Relationship, language and pre-understanding in the reflecting processes. *The Australian, New Zealand Journal of Family Therapy, 13*, 87–91.

Tom Andersen (1992). Interpersonal relationships, language and understanding. *Focus on the family, 1*(1992), 33–43.

Tom Andersen (1992). If research is a search for knowledge, what kind of knowledge is useful to search for relation to what? *AFTA newsletter, Spring 1992*, 33–36.

Tom Andersen (1992). A conversation with Tom Andersen. *Progress: Family Systems Research and Therapy, 1*, 3–24.

Tom Andersen (1992). *Videofilm:* "The reflecting process; informing others and forming self". *American Association for Marriage and Family Therapy*. Learning edge series.

1993

Tom Andersen (1993). See and hear, and be seen and heard. In S. Friedman (ed.), *The New Language of Change. Constructive Collaboration in Psychotherapy*. New York: Guilford Press.

Tom Andersen (1993). Comfortable interventions. In T. S. Nelson & T. S. Trepper (Eds.), *101 Interventions in Family Therapy*. New York: The Haworth Press.

Tom Andersen (1993). The illusion of the neutral therapist. Panel presentation at the 3rd Nordic Congress of Family Therapy 19–22 August Hotel Nyborg Strand Denmark. *Impuls 3*(1993), 59–67.

Tom Andersen (1993). *Clients and therapists as co-researchers to increase therapists' sensitivity*. First presented by the author at *the Lofoten conference* 22–25 June 1993 (Manuscript received privately by the author. Later published in Fokus, 4(95)).

Tom Andersen (1993). Commentary on Alex Reed's article: "The Reflecting Team in a Systemic Therapy Training Context- a Vehicle for Connected Teaching". *Human Systems: Journal of Systemic Consultation & Management, 4*, 229–230 (Reed's article pages 213–233).

Tom Andersen (1993). *Videofilm. A live consultation; reflecting processes* (Dialogue and dialogues about dialogues). Los Angeles Master work productions.

1994

Tom Andersen (1994). *Reflective processes. Conversations and conversations about conversations*. Copenhagen, Denmark: Dansk Psykologisk Forlag.

Tom Andersen (1994). Comments on two articles on research. *Focus on the Family, 2*(1994), 126–128.

Tom Andersen (1994). Reflecting processes. Shifting inner and outer talks where others are informed and one's self is formed. *The Australian, New Zealand Journal of Family Therapy, 15*, 10f.f.

Tom Andersen (1994). Stones and hands ("Stener og hender"). *Experimental activities for families, groups, teams and organisations*. Taos, New Mexico: The Taos inst. press. (Article obtained privately by the author. 2001).

Tom Andersen (1994). Power of knowledge and knowledge in language. *Feedback. The Magazine of Family Therapy Network of Ireland, 5*, 6–10.

Tom Andersen (1994). *Reflective processes*. Stockholm, Sweden: Mareld. New edition.

Tom Andersen (1994). "The Milan way - a big relief". *Newsletter of Centro Milanese di terapia del* famiglia (Comment: This seems to have been published only in Italian. Tom himself writes that he has sent it as - in press).

1995

Tom Andersen (1995). Reflecting processes; acts of informing and forming. You can borrow my eyes, but you must take them away from me. In S. Friedman (Ed.),

The Reflecting Team in Action: Collaborative Practice in Family Therapy. New York: Guilford Press.

Tom Andersen (1995). The pavilion a guesthouse. Alternatives in the psychiatric health service. *Utposten, 6*(1995), 278–287.

Tom Andersen (1995). *Language is powerful and might be dangerous.* Plenary talk at the 2nd World Family Therapy Congress, Guadalajara, Mexico October 25th to 29th. Manuscript received privately by the author, 2001.

Tom Andersen (1995). To be confirmed by being seen and heard. *Mental Health (Stockholm), 3*(1995), 206–215.

Tom Andersen (1995). Clients and therapists as co-researchers to increase therapists' sensitivity. *Focus on the Family, 4*(1995), 193–200.

Tom Andersen (1995). *Changes and developments in the field of systemic family therapy. Some thoughts.* Proceedings from The First European Congress of European Association of Multidisciplinary Practice for Mental Health Care of Children, Young People and Their Families (AESMEAF). Oslo Norway, June 30 to July 2.

Tom Andersen (1995). *In forming and forming aspects of reflecting processes.* Proceedings from The First European Congress of European Association of Multidisciplinary Practice for Mental Health care of Children, young people and their families (AESMEAF). Oslo Norway, June 30 to July 2.

1996

Tom Andersen (1996). *Reflective processes. Conversations and conversations about conversations* (2nd ed.). Copenhagen: Dansk psykologisk forlag.

Tom Andersen (1996). A few words about language. *Impulse, 4*(1996), 42–43.

Tom Andersen (1996). Research of treatment practice: What will or what should or what can such research be? A contribution to the debate. *Focus on the family, 1*(1996), 3–15.

Tom Andersen (1996). From vision to reality to new visions. Foreword in J. Seikkula, *Open dialogue.* Stocholm: Mareld.

Tom Andersen (1996). Language is not innocent. In F. W. Kaslow (Ed.), *Handbook of Relational Diagnosis and Dysfunctional Family Patterns.* New York: John Wiley & Sons.

1997

Tom Andersen (1997). The field of family therapy yesterday, today and tomorrow. Diversity, self-criticism and outlook - some thoughts. *Focus on the Family, 3–4*(1997), 152–153.

Tom Andersen (1997). Participatory practice and being-in-the-world. Some preliminary reflections. IN B. Ianssen (ed.), *Movement, life and change. In the footsteps of Aadel Bülow-Hansen.* Oslo: Cappelen Akademiske Forlag.

Tom Andersen (1997). Meeting with Mai in January 1996. IN B. Ianssen (ed.), *Movement, life and change. In the footsteps of Aadel Bülow-Hansen.* Oslo: Cappelen Akademiske Forlag.

Tom Andersen (1997). Interview with Tom. In E. Abrahamsen & G. Berglund *Creative conversations. Meetings with family therapists and their ideas*. Stockholm: Mareld.

Tom Andersen (1997). Miserere Nobis: A choir of small and big voices in despair. IN C. Smith & D. K. Nylund, *Narrative therapies with children and adolescents*. New York: Guilford Press.

Tom Andersen (1997). A book with a lot of sweet and strong touches and moves. Foreword in G. Fredman, *Death Talk*. London: Karnac Books.

1998

Tom Andersen (1998). One sentence of five lines about creating meaning: in perspective of relationship, prejudice and bewitchment preliminary attempts to explicate some thoughts that that everybody already have somehow thought of. *Human Systems: the journal of systemic consultation & management, 8*, 73–80.

Tom Andersen (1998). *The significance of expressions in treatment and research; Some preliminary formulations* (18 pages). Draft article. Received by the author.

Tom Andersen (1998). *The meaning of expressions in treatment and research; Some preliminary formulations* (51 pages). Draft article. Received by the author.

Tom Andersen (1998). *A travel letter: the journey back and forth between African dreams and African realities* (15 pages). Draft article. Received by the author.

Tom Andersen (1998). "The reversal of light and sound" From an interview with Tom Andersen. *Gecko, 2*, 5–9. Adelaide: Dulwich Centre Publications.

Tom Andersen (1998). Beautiful thoughts in beautiful surroundings. Report from NFFT's pre-Christmas seminar with Tom Andersen in gamle Logen. 2–3 December 1998. *Metaforum, 4*(1998), 4–7.

Tom Andersen (1998). What do you see if you look into that word? In F. N. Thomas & T. S. Nelson (eds.), *Tales from Family Therapy. Life - Changing Clinical Experiences*. New York: The Haworth Press.

1999

Tom Andersen (1999). A co-operation - by some called counselling. In M. H. Rønnestad & S. Reichelt (eds.), *Psychotherapy counselling*. Oslo: Tano Aschehoug.

Tom Andersen (1999). Travelling back and forth between African dreams and African realities. A travelogue. *Metaforum, 1*(1999), 4–10.

2000

Tom Andersen (2000). Reconciliation - is it always possible? A partly read talk on the 14th of June 2000 at the XII IFTA Family Therapy World Congress in Oslo. *Metaforum, 3–4*(2000), 14–17.

Tom Andersen (2000). Foreword in J. Seikkula, *Open conversations*. Oslo: Tano Aschehoug.

Tom Andersen (2000). Networking in the North Calotte. Afterword in R. Andresen (ed.), *Fellesskap og sammenhenger - Yrkeshjelpere i grupper, nettverk og organisasjoner*. Oslo: Gyldendal Akademisk.

2001

Tom Andersen (2001). *Kjellberg, E., Andersen, T. & Edwardsson, M. (eds.), *Man kan inte så noga veta ...: Child psychiatric investigations together with social services. Practice and research through reflective processes*. Stockholm: Mareld.

Tom Andersen (2001). Ethics before ontology: A few words. *Journal of Systemic Therapies, 20*(4), 11–13.

Tom Andersen (2001). *A co-operation called psychotherapy by some. Expressive bonds and meaningful expressions*. Draft article. Obtained by the author.

Tom Andersen (2001). *On Solidarity. Plenary Talk Budapest June 07.-02*. Manuscript. Provided by the author.

Tom Andersen (2001). *RUDAS: The Turkish bath in Budapest*. Draft article. Obtained by the author.

Tom Andersen (2001). *An ode to Harry*. Screenplay.

2002

Tom Andersen (2002). Blinding and deafening moments, and threatening futures: In the wake of 9.11. *Family Process, 41*(1), 11–14.

Tom Andersen (2002). A co-operation, by some called psychotherapy. Expressive bonds and meaningful expressions. In H. M. Rønnestad & A. von der Lippe, *The clinical interview* (pp. 314–333). Oslo: Gyldendal Akademisk.

2003

Tom Andersen (2003). The network context of network therapy. A story from the European Nordic North. Draft for a chapter in A. Lightburn & P. Session (eds.), *Community Based Clinical Practice*. New York: Oxford University Press. (Obtained privately by the author. This is cited later with reference to 2007 - in press).

Tom Andersen (2003). Vettre 2003 - Meeting with Tom Andersen: "An elderly man looks back on the professional choices he made on his walk" By Ingebriktsen H. *Metaforum 1*(2003), 18–20.

2004

Tom Andersen (2004). Families and the global crises and the global poverty. Plenary talk at IFTA's conference in Istanbul. *Metaforum, 3*(2004), 13–15.

Tom Andersen (2004). If your pain found a Voice what would it say? Psychotherapy as collaboration. *Human Systems: Journal of Systemic Consultation & Management, 15*(4), 213–226.

Tom Andersen (2004). Descriptions of reality. Vettre 2004. Workshop. Refereed by Ingebriktsen, H. *Metaforum, 2*(2004), 26–29. The June seminar in Tromsø 14–16 June 2004.

Tom Andersen (2004). "Appreciative, narrative and reflective language in consultation with Elspeth McAdam, England, Michael White, Australia and Tom Andersen Norway" Part 1. by Ingebriktsen H. *Metaforum, 3*(2004), 5–12. June seminar in Tromsø 14–16 June 2004.

Tom Andersen (2004). "Appreciative, narrative and reflective language in consultation with Elspeth McAdam, England, Michael White, Australia and Tom Andersen Norway" Part 2. by Ingebriktsen H. *Metaforum, 4*(2004), 14–21. The June seminar in Tromsø 14–16 June 2004.

2005

Tom Andersen (2005). *Reflective processes. Conversations and conversations about conversations* (3rd ed.). Copenhagen: Danish Psychological Publishers.

Tom Andersen (2005). Don't think, but see! Vettre 2005. Workshop. Referred to by H. C. Michaelsen, *Metaforum, 3*(2005), 6–8.

Tom Andersen (2004). Two vignettes. 1: Sixty - two years after. *Metaforum, 3*(2005), 22–25.

2006

Tom Andersen (2006). Experiences and challenges in relationship work. Systemic café 6 June. Referenced by H. Ingebriktsen, *Metaforum, 3*(2006), 5–9.

Tom Andersen (2006). Crossroads. Tom Andersen in conversation with Per Jensen. By P. Jensen, *Focus on the Family, 3*(2006), 163–173.

Tom Andersen (2006). Reflective conversations; my version. In H. Eliassen & J. Seikkula (eds.), *Reflective Processes in Practice*. Oslo: Universitetsforlaget.

Tom Andersen (2006). Foreword in S. Baum & H. Lynggaard, *Intellectual Disabilities: A Systemic Approach*. Karnac Books.

Tom Andersen (2006). What we investigate, we do together. In E. Abrahamsson & G. Berglund, *Psykoterapins förnyare - samtal om systemisk förändringsarbete*. Stockholm: Mareld.

Tom Andersen (2006). Elpeth McAdam, Michael White and Tom Andersen "Tromsø, June 2004". In E. Abrahamsson & G. Berglund, *Psykoterapins förnyare - samtal om systemisk förändringsarbete*. Stockholm: Mareld.

2007

Tom Andersen (2007). Human Participating: Human "being" is the step for human "becoming" in the next step. In H. Anderson & D. Gehart (Eds.), *Collaborative Therapy Relationships and Conversations that Make a Difference*. London: Routledge.

Tom Andersen (2007). Crossroads. In H. Andersen & P. Jensen (Eds.), *Innovations in Reflecting Processes* (pp. 158–174). London: Karnac.

Tom Andersen (2012). Words - universes travelling by. In T. Malinen, S. J. Cooper & F. N. Thomas, *Masters of Narrative and Collaborative Therapies: The Voices of Andersen, Anderson and White*. London: Routledge.

DVDs:

1997: Staff meeting at BUP Tromsø "The bewitchment of language". Private ownership.

2005: "Open conversations - don't talk about the unspeakable". Interview with Professor Tom Andersen and Professor Jaakko Seikkula. Knowledge Centre for Social Psychiatry ANTV; Mediehuset Århus.

2006: "Test recording for a video". Unedited raw material. Private property.

2007: "Att finna sina egna ord". Uppsala County Council (Swedish, English and Spanish subtitles).

2008: "Tom Andersen and John Shotter in joint action" London UK Conference 2003. With additional material in honour of the late Tom Andersen. KCC International in association with Victory Video. UK.

Annet:

1996: Dialogue and reflection. *Festschrift to Professor Tom Andersen on his 60th birthday*. ISM publication series, no. 35. University of Tromsø, Department of Public Health.

On 15 May 2007, Tom dies in an accident. Since then, several books have been published about the work he has done.

Focus on the family, 3(2007) is a commemorative issue.

Anderson, H. & Jensen, P. (eds.) (2007). *Innovations in the reflecting process. The inspiration of Tom Andersen*. London: Karnac.

In Norwegian (2008). *Inspiration. Tom Andersen and reflective processes*. Oslo: Gyldendal Akademisk.

Malinen, T., Cooper, S. J. & Thomas, F. N. (2011). *Masters of Narrative and Collaborative Therapies. The Voices of Andersen, Anderson and White*. New York: Routledge.

Afterword

Can a book on reflecting teams and reflecting processes tell us something important about the practice of psychotherapy today? Certainly, when the three of us started the work of putting together this book, we were clear about our opinion on this question. By putting this book together, the obvious answer is "yes", but why? To close this book by answering this question, it is necessary to visit the Norwegian contemporary context of psychotherapy. After more or less 25 years with the concept of evidence-based practice as the developing focus of psychotherapy research and practice, something is happening. One manner of looking at the "evidence movement" in psychotherapy is through the idea that if we know about effects on the group level of a diagnostic category, this speaks to what will be effective for the single person or family. At the same time, we know from this group-based research, through the use of the randomised controlled trial, that not only is there a part of the diagnostic group that is helped, but it is also evident that some are not helped by the investigated method and some actually get worse. Although the concept of evidence-based practice has been modified to include both the skills and knowledge of the therapist and the characteristics, cultural backgrounds and preferences of the patient and the family, questions can be raised if this is enough to secure an ethical and helpful practice for the patient and the family.

What we see in our context is that the use of evidence-based methods and practices demands selection. Since we know some are not helped, we need to assess every person and judge if the person is to be included in the method used or not. Concepts like patient-fitted and patient-adapted treatment are moving into the centre of the debate about how to secure the aim of fitting the single person and family to the best method for them. Our health authorities are more and more demanding that the methods used should be evidence-based; at the same time, no guidelines are developed for how to meet those who are not fit for the method. We all agree that the future is to tailor treatment to the patient and family. The question is how to do this. The keyword in the traditional field of psychotherapy research and practice in Norway is to pursue an idea of identifying subgroups within diagnostic categories and a modified evidence-based, theory-specific method into which the single person and family belonging to the subgroup can be fitted. Within a diagnostic group, for instance eating disorders, it makes a difference how such a method is used if the person has experienced sexual abuse or not. With this, we see a search for subgroups and subgroups of subgroups of persons that can be fitted to the method. The solution is to select patients that fit the subgroup and a modified theory-specific method. With this, it follows that the other side of the coin is the exclusion of those who cannot be fitted to the subgroup and its therapeutic method. So, the question is still: what about those who fall outside the parameters of the subgroups. What about the outliers?

It is here that we find another solution and manner of thinking in the work of the Tromsø group and Tom Andersen. It is our assertion that the idea of patient-adapted methods and practices actually had one of its starting points when the Tromsø group turned on light and sound in the one-way mirror room. Contemporary, mainstream psychotherapy seems finally to have reached the point that the Tromsø group and Tom Andersen reached over 40 years ago. How come this assertion?

In the book you are holding in your hand, Tom Andersen describes how working in a traditional Milano-systemic way, where the therapists left the room and talked about the family with their colleagues behind the mirror was experienced as extremely uncomfortable. At some point, this distress among the therapists led to a radical move. The light and sound were turned on, and the family was invited to listen to the conversations behind the mirror between the therapists and then comment on these conversations. This was a radical move. Why radical? For us, because it included the family directly in the therapeutic work. The family`s responses, thoughts and feedback had to be taken seriously, and with that, the family became a participant in the design of the therapeutic processes. It also meant an increased awareness and sensitivity among the therapists regarding their relational forms and contributions. This put the therapeutic relationship on the agenda, together with collaboration and an emphasis on egalitarian ways of working. It is no coincidence that the concepts of peace work and democracy have a place in this book. A decisive question of practice became how to conduct conversations that enabled good relational experiences for the family and a functioning collaboration for both the family and the therapists. This again has been part of opening up the field of family therapy to dialogical and narrative forms of practice. Last but not least, it became clear that helpful therapy meant creating a process that suited and fit the context, life experience and history of the family. Treatment had to be fitted to the family. This fitting implies an alternative approach to patient- and family-adapted treatments. It is no longer a question of finding the persons who fit a subgroup that has a corresponding, theory-specific, evidence-based method that is helpful for a specific diagnostic subgroup. It is about therapist change.

For this editor group, this perspective has followed us throughout our careers. Magnus, as part of the Tromsø group, has specifically pursued this by working to establish medication-free treatments for persons experiencing serious mental problems. Bengt has pursued the ideas of recovery orientation within mental health services and the consequences it has for practice. Rolf has pursued the ideas of patient-focused research and the use of feedback from families in making treatment, together with the families, that is fitted to their needs and goals. Running through this, based on the ideas that were developed in Tromsø and the work with reflecting teams and processes, it is not about fitting the patient and family into a diagnostic subgroup. It is all about therapist change. When therapists and their methods and practices are not helpful, therapists need to change their way of working. This change must be governed by the responses, participation and collaboration of the family. For us, the power of the family therapy practices that the Tromsø group and Tom Andersen initiated was to take Gregory Bateson seriously in putting difference (that makes a difference) at the centre stage of family therapy. As living entities, as human beings, we are similar in that we are all different, and these differences, small or big, will make a difference in how therapy is done. No membership in a subgroup or subgroup of subgroups will change this fact. We need to give priority to difference over similarity. We need to make therapy an idiosyncratic and patient-fitted event in the life of people, and let similarities and generalisations at best be a starting point for therapeutic work. At worst, it can become a de-individualised and de-contextualised practice of mental health care that will increasingly become inhuman and undemocratic. For us, this is the legacy of Tom Andersen and the Tromsø group. In our contemporary situation, this voice needs to be heard and strengthened. We therefore believe in this book and the ideas and practices that it brings forth.

Index

Note: *Italic* page numbers refer to figures and page numbers followed by 'n' refer to notes.

"aesthetics" *versus* "pragmatics" 38
all in one room 160
Anderson, H. 3, 7, 48, 77, 79–83; "Human Systems as Linguistic Systems: Preliminary and Evolving Ideas about the Implications for Clinical Theory" 81–82

Bakhtin, M. 139
balance 40–41
Bateson, G. 33, 35–39, 45, 48, 83, 159; *Mind and Nature* 36, 158
beating 168–169
being "depressed" 14
bodily knowledge 143
body movements 40, 41
Boscolo, L. 32, 77
both-and attitude 3, 62, 71
Bowen, M. 48
Braatøy, T. 42, 44
Bråten, S. 77
breathing: movements 46; for muscle tension 43, 45–47
Bülow-Hansen, A. 2–4, 8, 27, 42, 44, 47, 51

Cecchin, G. 2, 32, 77
"change comes from within" 60–61
chronic treatment failures 48
circularity 33, 36–37
coercion 2, 10, 61, 163
collaboration 131–138
colonisation 125–126
constructivism 39; radical 78
contextual perspective 57–58
counselling exercise 179–180
crabbing 168–169
cybernetics 7, 37; epistemology 79; language 37, 83; second-order 77–80, 83; thinking 48

Dell, P. 48
democracy 2
domination 125–126
"double bind" theory 159

either-or attitude 3, 62, 71
empiricism 82
entropy 36
epistemology 35–39, 80, 157; cybernetic 79
ethics 66–67
everyday language 55–57, 105, 110, 120
exhalation (expiration) 46
expert language 55–57, 105, 120
expressions: and impressions, relationship between 4; increased awareness of 163–166; meanings of, in treatment and research 104–127; power of 91–103; without words 166–170

family therapy 31; phases of 32–33; structural 48; systems theory-oriented 7, 26
feelings within feelings 169–170
Flåm, A. M. 77
Frankfurt, M. 101
fundamental beliefs 106, 127

Gadamer, H.-G. 106
Galveston group 77, 78
Gergen, K. 82, 83

Goolishian, H. 3, 7, 38, 47–49, 51, 65, 77, 79–83, 137, 138, 179; on expression 108; "Human Systems as Linguistic Systems: Preliminary and Evolving Ideas about the Implications for Clinical Theory" 81–82
Goolishian School of Therapy, The 46
"Greek Kitchen in the Arctic, A" seminar, Sulitjelma (1988) 76–84
group counselling 161
group therapy 161

Hald, M.: as an intern 22–23; as a general practitioner 23–24; professional development 31–49; as a psychiatric hospital doctor 24–25; as a university employee 26; *see also individual entries*
Haley, J. 2, 31, 38, 48
Heidegger, M. 106
hermeneutic circle 106–107, *107*, *109*, *112–114*
Hoffman, L. 2, 48, 77
homeostasis 38
Hudson, H. 31
human beings 67–68
"Human Systems as Linguistic Systems: Preliminary and Evolving Ideas about the Implications for Clinical Theory" (Goolishian and Anderson) 81–82

impression: appeal to reason 121–122; and expression, relationship between 4; meaning of 110–121
imprisoned men, conversations with 143–147
individual perspective 57–58
inhalation (inspiration) 46
interactional therapy 48
intervention-oriented therapy 39

Jackson, D.: *Pragmatics of Human Communication* 38
Jensen, P.: "Solidarity" 4–5
Josiah Macy group 37

kindness 84
King, M. L.: on peace 2
Kvale, S. 123

labelling 111
language 179–182; assumptions about 177–179; basic ideas about 107–110; community 120; cybernetic 37, 83; everyday 55–57, 105, 110, 120; expert 55–57, 105, 120; pathological 25, 55, 57; systems 83
"let them tell us what they want us to hear" 64–65
Levinas, E. 45–46
Lichtenberg, G. C. 35
linearity 33–34, 36
linguistic formulations 120
live consultations, at conferences 161–162
love 80

MacGregor, R. 47
making distinctions 118–119
marginalisation 125–126
market fundamentalism 20
Martino, E. 79
Martino, S. 79
Maturana, H. 9, 38–39, 48, 77–80; on love 80
mental health care 2, 6, 10, 163, 201
midstream 51–52
Milan group 2, 32, 34, 38, 77
Milan method 7
militant fundamentalism 20
mind: definition of 37, 158
Mind and Nature (Bateson) 36, 158
Minuchin, S. 2, 31, 48
MIT *see* Multiple Impact Therapy (MIT)
Morgan, G. 125
Multiple Impact Therapy (MIT) 47–48
muscle tension 42–45; breathing for 43, 45–47; release of 43; stretching for 43

naming 111–113
negentropy 36
networking 26–27, 161
network meetings 153–154
normality 32
Norwegian Association for Family Therapy 9

objective reality 82
observation 65–66
onion theory 82, 83
ontology 45, 66–67
open dialogue 62–64, 73, 139–141
oppression 2, 50
Øvreberg, G. 2, 8, 27, 40–42; on balance 40–41; on body movements 40

Palo Alto Group 48
participation 65–66, 147–150

Participatory Action Research 180
pathological language 25, 55, 57
peace 2
Penn, P. 2, 101, 147–150
perseverance 50–51, 139–141
perturbation 39
Philosophical Investigations (Wittgenstein) 117
Pragmatics of Human Communication (Watzlawick, Jackson & Beavin) 38
"pragmatics" *versus* "aesthetics" 38
Prigogine, I. 48
prioritisation 125–126
problematic situation (mental health): characterisation of 85–86; description of 85; finding 84–85; solutions, finding 86–87
problem-created system 179
psychiatry *see* mental health care
psychodynamic theories 31
psychomotor physiotherapy 44
Psychosis Network 153
"Psychotherapies for the Next Millennium" conference (1991) 83
psychotic crisis 116, 117, 141

radical constructivism 78
reality 68–70
reflective conversations 172–176; about process 181–182; approaches in 159–166; assumptions about language 177–179; assumptions about living people 177; assumptions about reality 176; elements of 157–159; meeting with authorities 162–163; team's reflections 173–174; therapeutic conversations 180–181; translation 171
reflective teams 71–87; conversation 73–75; "Greek Kitchen in the Arctic, A" seminar, Sulitjelma (1988) 76–84; guidelines for 75–76; solution to mental health problem 84–87
Reichelt, E. 111, 125–126
research: definition of 122; and practice, difference between 122
Ricoeur, P. 105
Ritchie, A. 47
Robin Hood institute (earlier Galveston Family Institute) 48
Rorty, R. 49

Sartre, J.-P. 78
schizogenesis 37
second-order cybernetics 77–80, 83
Seikkula, J. 3, 124, 139
self: evolving 39; forming 39; transforming 39
Shotter, J. 3, 87n1
Smedslund, J. 83
smiles/laughs 167–168
social constructionism 35, 82, 158
sociology of illness 53, 54
solidarity 4–5, 20, 50, 59, 60
solution-oriented therapy 39
staff meetings 161
Steier, F. 77, 79
strategic therapy 31, 32, 48
stretching, for muscle tension 43
structural family therapy 48
structural therapy 31, 32
structure-oriented therapy 39
suitably unusual 11, 39, 45, 65, 132
systemic family therapy 7
systemic legacy 35–39
systems theory 7, 26
systems theory-oriented family therapy 26

Talberg, P. 83
theory and practice 58–60
therapeutic meetings, conversation in 156–159, 180–181
Tromsø group 77, 78, 83

Varela, F. 48
Vedeler, A. H. 87n1
von Foerster, H. 77–79
von Glasersfeld, E. 77, 78
Vygotsky, L. 148

Wagner, J. 143, 144
Watzlawick, P.: *Pragmatics of Human Communication* 38
"we want them to tell us what we want to hear" 64–65
Whitaker, C. 48
Wittgenstein, L. 80, 104, 111, 115, 116; *Philosophical Investigations* 117
words, power of 91–103
working inside/outside, in psychiatric hospitals 54–55
write and speak 61–62

For Product Safety Concerns and Information please contact our EU
representative GPSR@taylorandfrancis.com
Taylor & Francis Verlag GmbH, Kaufingerstraße 24, 80331 München, Germany

www.ingramcontent.com/pod-product-compliance
Ingram Content Group UK Ltd.
Pitfield, Milton Keynes, MK11 3LW, UK
UKHW020007200926
475702UK00015B/2511

* 9 7 8 1 0 3 2 4 1 3 6 4 8 *